Lecture Notes
Haematology

AUTHORED BY,

N.C. Hughes-Jones
DM, PhD, MA, FRCP, FRS
Former Member of the Scientific Staff
Medical Research Council's Molecular Immunopathology Unit, and of
the Department of Pathology, University of Cambridge

S.N. Wickramasinghe
ScD, PhD, MB, BS, FRCPath, FRCP, FIBiol
Emeritus Professor of Haematology
Imperial College, University of London;
Visiting Professor of Haematology
University of Oxford;
Honorary Consultant Haematologist
St Mary's NHS Trust, London

C.S.R. Hatton
FRCP, FRCPath
Consultant Haematologist
Department of Haematology
The John Radcliffe Hospital
Oxford

Eighth Edition

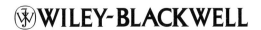
WILEY-BLACKWELL

This edition first published 1970, © 1973, 1979, 1984, 1991, 1996, 2004, 2009 by N.C. Hughes-Jones, S.N. Wickramasinghe, C.S.R. Hatton

Blackwell Publishing was acquired by John Wiley & Sons in February 2007. Blackwell's publishing program has been merged with Wiley's global Scientific, Technical and Medical business to form Wiley-Blackwell.

Registered office: John Wiley & Sons Ltd, The Atrium, Southern Gate, Chichester, West Sussex, PO19 8SQ, UK

Editorial offices: 9600 Garsington Road, Oxford, OX4 2DQ, UK
                         The Atrium, Southern Gate, Chichester, West Sussex, PO19 8SQ, UK
                         111 River Street, Hoboken, NJ 07030-5774, USA

For details of our global editorial offices, for customer services and for information about how to apply for permission to reuse the copyright material in this book please see our website at www.wiley.com/wiley-blackwell

Library of Congress Cataloging-in-Publication Data

Lecture notes. Haematology / N.C. Hughes-Jones, S.N. Wickramasinghe, C.S.R. Hatton. — 8th ed.
      p. ; cm.
    Rev. ed. of: Lecture notes on haematology / N.C. Hughes-Jones, S.N. Wickramasinghe, C.S.R. Hatton. 7th ed. 2004.
    Includes bibliographical references and index.
    ISBN 978-1-4051-8050-4
    1. Blood—Diseases—Outlines, syllabi, etc. I. Hughes-Jones, N.C. (Nevin Campbell) II. Wickramasinghe, S.N.
  III. Hatton, C.S.R. FRCP. IV. Hughes-Jones, N.C. (Nevin Campbell). Lecture notes
on haematology. V. Title: Haematology.
    [DNLM: 1. Hematologic Diseases. WH 120 L471 2008]

    RC636.H83 2008
    616.1'5—dc22

                                                                                                          2008003865

ISBN: 978-1-4051-8050-4

A catalogue record for this book is available from the British Library.

Set in 8/12 pt Stone Serif by Charon Tec Ltd., A Macmillan Company (www.macmillan solutions.com)

Printed & bound in Singapore by Utopia Press Pte Ltd
1   2009

Contents

Preface to the First Edition

These lecture notes are designed to supply the basic knowledge of both the clinical and laboratory aspects of haematological diseases and blood transfusion. The content is broadly similar to that of the course given to medical students by the Department of Haematology at St. Mary's Hospital Medical School. References have been cited so that those who need to extend their knowledge in any particular field can do so. Most of the journals and books that are mentioned are those commonly found in every library.

At the end of each chapter I have supplied learning objectives in studying each disease. There are two main purposes in these objectives. First, they facilitate the learning process, since the process of acquisition, retention, and recall of data is greatly helped if the facts and concepts are centred around a particular objective. Secondly, many objectives are closely related to the practical problems encountered in the diagnosis and treatment of patients. For instance, the following objectives: "to understand the method of differentiation of megaloblastic anaemia due to vitamin B_{12} deficiency from that due to folate deficiency" and "to understand the basis for the differentiation of leukaemia into acute and chronic forms based on the clinical picture and on the peripheral blood findings" are practical problems encountered frequently in the haematology laboratory. A point of more immediate interest to the undergraduate is that examiners setting either multiple choice or essay questions will be searching for the same knowledge that is required in answering the objectives.

I should like to thank Prof. P.L. Mollison, Dr. P. Barkhan, Dr. I. Chanarin, Dr. G.J. Jenkins, and Dr. M.S. Rose for their criticism and helpful suggestions during the preparation of the manuscript and Mrs. Inge Barnett for typing the several drafts and final typescript.

N.C. Hughes-Jones

Preface to the Eighth Edition

Since the publication of the last edition in 2004, there have been significant advances in a number of areas of haematology. In this edition, we have updated all of the chapters, ensuring that only core knowledge required by medical students is included. As in previous editions each chapter begins with a section on 'Objectives' in order to facilitate learning and revision and non-core information is in smaller type. As before, clinical and haematological features of a disease are explained in terms of pathophysiology and, when known, the underlying genetic defect or defects and secondary molecular abnormalities.

N.C. Hughes-Jones
S.N. Wickramasinghe
C.S.R. Hatton

Chapter 1

Normal Haemoglobin, Blood Cells and Haemopoiesis

Learning objectives

- To have a basic understanding of the structure and functions of the haemoglobin molecule.
- To know about the general features of globin genes — their location, structure, transcription and translation.
- To be able to identify the various types of normal blood cells in photographs.
- To know the functions, concentration and lifespan of various types of blood cell.
- To understand the concept of a stem cell.
- To understand how blood cells are produced from pluripotent haemopoietic stem cells and how haemopoiesis is regulated.
- To be able to identify erythroblasts, neutrophil precursors and megakaryocytes in photographs.
- To be aware of differences in the sites of haemopoiesis during human development and the reappearance of extramedullary haemopoiesis in some haematological disorders.

Normal haemoglobin and its synthesis

Structure and function

Normal human haemoglobins (Hbs) are tetramers consisting of two pairs of unlike globin chains;

Lecture Notes: Haematology, by NC Hughes-Jones, SN Wickramsinghe, CSR Hatton © 2008 Blackwell Publishing, ISBN: 9781405180504

each of the four chains is associated with one haem group located within a hydrophobic crevice. In adult Hbs, α-chains are associated mainly with β-chains (HbA; $\alpha_2\beta_2$) and to a much lesser extent with δ-chains (HbA$_2$; $\alpha_2\delta_2$). In fetal Hb, α-chains are associated with γ-chains (HbF; $\alpha_2\gamma_2$). In the embryonic Hbs, ζ-chains are associated with ε-chains (Hb Gower 1; $\zeta_2\varepsilon_2$) or γ-chains (Hb Portland; $\zeta_2\gamma_2$) and α-chains are associated with ε-chains (Hb Gower 2; $\alpha_2\varepsilon_2$). There are two types of γ-chains in HbF which differ only in the amino acid at position 136, which may be glycine ($^G\gamma$-chains) or alanine ($^A\gamma$-chains).

When the percentage O_2 saturation of Hb at various O_2 tensions (in mmHg) is determined in the laboratory and the two values are plotted against each other, a sigmoid O_2 dissociation (O_2 affinity) curve is obtained (Fig. 1.1). This is because the binding of one O_2 molecule to the haem group on one globin chain of the tetrameric Hb molecule promotes the binding of the next O_2 molecule to the haem group on another globin chain. This haem–haem interaction results from a small shape change in the molecule that occurs when O_2 combines with haem. In the deoxygenated state, the two β-chains are separated slightly, such that one molecule of 2,3-diphosphoglycerate (2,3-DPG) can enter the Hb molecule and bind to the β-chains; in the oxygenated state, the 2,3-DPG is ejected. The partial pressure of O_2 at which normal Hb is half saturated with O_2 (P_{50}) is 26 mmHg

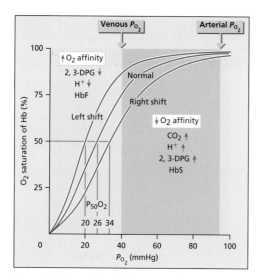

Figure 1.1 Oxygen dissociation curves of human blood.

(at pH 7.4, 37°C). *In vivo*, exchange of O_2 normally occurs between a P_{O_2} of 95 mmHg (95% saturation) in arterial blood and a P_{O_2} of 40 mmHg (70% saturation) in venous blood.

The O_2 affinity of Hb is decreased (the O_2 dissociation curve is shifted to the right) by an increase in the amount of CO_2 in the blood (Bohr effect). The CO_2 generates hydrogen ions by reacting with water, and the reduced O_2 affinity results from the combination of hydrogen ions with deoxyhaemoglobin; these hydrogen ions are released when Hb is oxygenated. Thus the Bohr effect facilitates the release of O_2 in tissues and the unloading of CO_2 in the lungs. A second mechanism by which CO_2 generated in the tissues decreases the O_2 affinity of Hb (i.e. facilitates the release of O_2) is by reacting with the amino groups of the α-globin chains to form carbamates. When Hb combines with O_2 in the alveoli, this CO_2 is released.

The O_2 affinity of Hb is increased by a decrease in 2,3-DPG levels as occurs in stored blood, and decreased by an increase in 2,3-DPG levels as occurs in hypoxia. The O_2 affinity of HbF is higher than that of HbA because γ-chains bind to 2,3-DPG more weakly than β-chains. The high affinity of HbF facilitates O_2 transport from the mother to the fetus. O_2 affinity is decreased

in sickle cell anaemia and also by an increase in body temperature (e.g. during fever).

Synthesis

The genes for the ε-, $^{G}\gamma$-, $^{A}\gamma$-, δ- and β-chains are found in this order (5' to 3') in a linked cluster on chromosome 11. The α gene is duplicated so that there are two α genes close to the ζ gene on chromosome 16 in the linkage order ζ, α_2, α_1 (5' to 3'). Interestingly, in both chromosomes 11 and 16, the genes are arranged in the order in which they are switched on during intrauterine life.

There are a number of conserved sequences in the upstream flanking regions of the globin genes. Such sequences are involved in the regulation of globin gene expression and are known as promoters. In addition, there are other local regulatory elements termed enhancers situated at various distances either 5' or 3' to the gene. The promoters are involved in the attachment and correct positioning of the transcription initiation complex, which includes RNA polymerase (the enzyme involved in mRNA synthesis). The globin gene promoters and enhancers are recognized by non-specific (ubiquitous) transcription factors, erythroid tissue-specific transcription factors such as GATA-1, GATA-2 and erythroid Krüppel-like factors (EKLF), and developmental stage-specific transcription factors. Expression of genes in the entire β-globin gene cluster is influenced by a remote regulatory region known as the β-locus control region (β-LCR), which is situated upstream of the ε gene. Expression of genes in the entire α-globin gene cluster is controlled by a regulatory element known as HS-40 located upstream of the ζ gene.

Each globin gene contains two non-coding regions, also known as intervening sequences (IVSs) or introns (i.e. regions that are not represented in the mature mRNA) and three coding regions or exons (Fig. 1.2). The initial mRNA transcript (mRNA precursor) is large and complementary to all regions (coding and non-coding) of the globin gene, but the regions complementary to the base sequences of the introns are soon removed by excision and ligation (spliced) and are absent in the mature mRNA. Within the nucleus,

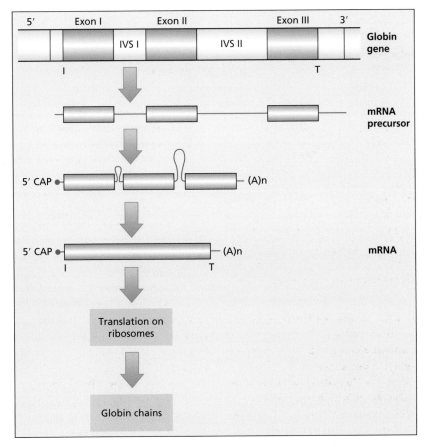

Figure 1.2 Expression of globin genes. *Notes*: IVS — intervening sequence; I — initiator codon; T — termination codon; (A)n — polyadenylation site; 5′ CAP — structure containing 7-methyl guanosine.

the mRNA is modified at the 5′ end by the formation of a CAP structure and is stabilized by polyadenylation at the 3′ end. The mature mRNA enters the cytoplasm and attaches to ribosomes on which globin chain synthesis (translation) occurs.

Blood cells

Morphology

On Romanowsky-stained blood smears, normal erythrocytes appear as red, anucleate cells with circular outlines and have diameters between 6.7 and 7.7 μm (mean 7.2 μm). Blood-cell morphology should be assessed in a region of the blood smear in which only occasional red cells overlap. In such

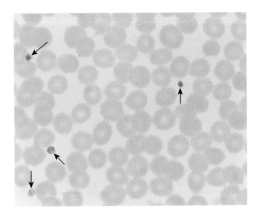

Figure 1.3 Smear of normal peripheral venous blood. The red cells are round and do not vary greatly in size. They are well filled with haemoglobin; the central area of pallor is small. A few platelets (arrowed) are also present.

Table 1.1 Morphology of normal white cells in Romanowsky-stained smears of peripheral blood.

| Cell type | Cell size (μm) | Cytoplasm | | Granules | Nucleus |
		Colour	Ratio of cytoplasmic volume to nuclear volume		
Neutrophil granulocytes	9–15	Slightly pink	High	Numerous, very fine, faint purple	Usually two to five segments
Eosinophil granulocytes	12–17	Pale blue	High	Many, large and rounded, reddish-orange	Usually two segments
Basophil granulocytes	10–14		High	Several, large and rounded, dark purplish-black	Usually two segments, granules overlie nucleus
Monocytes	15–30	Pale greyish-blue, cytoplasmic vacuoles may be seen	Moderately high or high	Variable number, fine, purplish-red	Various shapes (rounded, C- or U-shaped, lobulated), skein-like or lacy chromatin
Lymphocytes	7–12 (small lymphocytes)	Pale blue	Low or very low	Few, fine purplish-red	Rounded with large clumps of condensed chromatin
	12–16 (large lymphocytes)	Pale blue	Higher	Several, coarser, purplish-red	Less condensation of chromatin

a region, each red cell (which is biconcave in shape) has a central area of pallor whose diameter is about a third of the red cell diameter (Fig. 1.3).

In addition to red cells, blood smears contain platelets and various types of white cell. On average, the ratio between red cells, platelets and leucocytes is 700:40:1. The platelets are small anucleate cells, about 2–3 μm in diameter (Fig. 1.3). They stain light blue and contain a number of small azurophilic granules, which are often concentrated at the centre. The important features of the morphology of normal leucocytes are summarized in Table 1.1. Neutrophil, eosinophil and basophil granulocytes (Fig. 1.4) are also described as polymorphonuclear leucocytes or polymorphs: the two or more nuclear masses in each cell are joined in series by fine strands of nuclear chromatin. Normally, the proportion of neutrophil polymorphs with five or more nuclear segments is 3% or less. A monocyte is shown in Fig. 1.4(c). Small lymphocytes (Fig. 1.5) account for about 90% of lymphocytes in the blood; large lymphocytes for the remaining 10%. Many of the large lymphocytes contain several prominent purplish-red granules in their cytoplasm (Fig. 1.6).

Number and lifespan

The reference ranges for concentrations of various types of blood cell in adults are given in Table 1.2, together with data on their lifespan in the blood. Ranges for the Hb and packed cell volume (PCV) in healthy individuals are given on p. 16. Normal red cells circulate for 110–120 days and at the end of their lifespan are phagocytosed in the bone marrow, spleen, and liver by macrophages

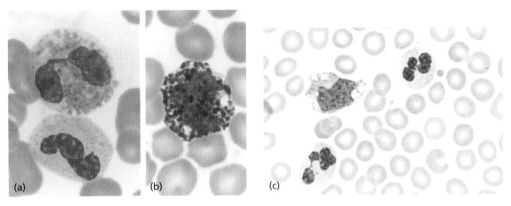

Figure 1.4 Smear of normal peripheral venous blood: (a) neutrophil granulocyte and eosinophil granulocyte; (b) basophil granulocyte; and (c) monocyte and two neutrophil granulocytes — the monocyte has a pale, greyish-blue vacuolated cytoplasm. Figure (c) is at a lower magnification than (a) and (b).

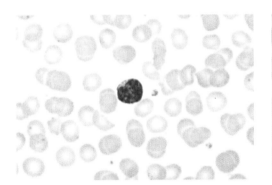

Figure 1.5 A small lymphocyte in a normal blood smear.

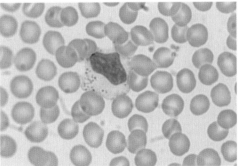

Figure 1.6 Large lymphocyte with several azurophilic cytoplasmic granules. Large granular lymphocytes (LGLs) include cytotoxic T cells and natural killer (NK) cells (p. 7). *Source*: Courtesy of Dr. Barbara Bain.

Table 1.2 Ninety-five percent reference limits for the concentrations of various types of circulating blood cell in adults and their lifespan in the blood.

Cell type	Reference range (95% reference limits)	Lifespan in blood
Red cells	Males 4.4–5.8 × 10^{12}/L	110–120 days
	Females 4.1–5.2 × 10^{12}/L	
White cells (leucocytes)	4.0–11.0 × 10^9/L*	
Neutrophil granulocytes	1.5–7.5 × 10^9/L*	$t_{1/2}$ approx. 7 h
Eosinophil granulocytes	0.02–0.60 × 10^9/L	$t_{1/2}$ approx. 6 h
Basophil granulocytes	0.01–0.15 × 10^9/L	
Monocytes	0.2–0.8 × 10^9/L	$t_{1/2}$ approx. 70 h
Lymphocytes	1.2–3.5 × 10^9/L	
Platelets	160–450 × 10^9/L	9–12 days

Note: *Applies to Caucasians.

Table 1.3 The main functions of blood cells.

Type of cell	Main functions
Red blood cells (erythrocytes)	Transport O_2 from lungs to tissues; transport CO_2 from tissues to lungs (see p. 1)
Neutrophil granulocytes	Chemotaxis, phagocytosis, killing of phagocytosed bacteria
Eosinophil granulocytes	All neutrophil functions listed above, effector cells for antibody-dependent damage to metazoal parasites, regulate immediate-type hypersensitivity reactions (inactivate histamine and leukotrienes released by basophils and mast cells)
Basophil granulocytes	Mediate immediate-type hypersensitivity (IgE-coated basophils react with specific antigen and release histamine and leukotrienes), modulate inflammatory responses by releasing heparin and proteases
Monocytes (and macrophages*)	Chemotaxis, phagocytosis, killing of some microorganisms, antigen presentation, release of IL-1 and TNF which stimulate bone marrow stromal cells to produce GM-CSF, G-CSF, M-CSF, and IL-6 (p. 15)
Platelets	Adhere to subendothelial connective tissue, participate in blood clotting (see p. 147)
Lymphocytes	Involved in immune responses and production of haemopoietic growth factors (p. 7)

Note: *Macrophages are tissue cells derived from monocytes.

(a component of the reticuloendothelial system). The neutrophil granulocytes in the blood are distributed between a marginated granulocyte pool (consisting of cells that are loosely attached to the endothelial lining of small venules) and a circulating granulocyte pool. There is a continuous exchange of cells between these two pools and in healthy subjects, the circulating granulocyte pool accounts for between 16% and 99% (average, 44%) of all blood granulocytes. When cell counts are determined on samples of peripheral venous blood, only the circulating granulocytes are being studied. In healthy Caucasian adults, the reference range for the absolute neutrophil count is $1.5–7.5 \times 10^9$/L. The lower limit for the reference range is lower in healthy blacks, being about 1.0×10^9/L. Neutrophil granulocytes leave the circulation exponentially, with an average $t_{1/2}$ of about 7h, and probably survive in tissues and secretions for about another 30h.

Lymphocytes continuously recirculate between the blood and lymphatic system. They leave the blood between the endothelial cells of the postcapillary venules of lymph nodes, migrate through the lymph node into efferent lymphatics and re-enter the blood via the thoracic duct. The majority of human lymphocytes are long-lived, with average lifespans of 4–5 years and maximum lifespans of greater than 20 years. The short-lived lymphocytes survive for about 3 days.

Functions

The main functions of blood cells are summarized in Table 1.3. More details of platelet function are given on p. 147.

Neutrophils and monocytes

Monocytes are the precursors of tissue macrophages. Phagocytosis of microorganisms and cells coated with antibody (with their exposed Fc fragments) and complement (especially C3b) occurs via binding to Fc and C3b receptors on the surface of neutrophils, monocytes and macrophages. Bacteria and fungi that are not antibody coated are phagocytosed after binding to mannose receptors on the phagocyte surface. The killing of phagocytosed microorganisms involves superoxide (O_2^-)-dependent and O_2-independent mechanisms.

The superoxide-dependent microbicidal agents include H_2O_2, hypochlorous acid, chloramines and hydroxyl radicals ($OH^\bullet$). Superoxide (O_2^-) is produced by neutrophils and some γ-interferon-stimulated macrophages during the respiratory burst which follows their activation and lasts from a few seconds to 15 min. The generation of O_2^- results from the reduction of O_2 by NADPH, which is catalysed by NADPH oxidase, one component of which is membrane-bound flavocytochrome b_{558}. The O_2^- undergoes dismutation to O_2 and H_2O_2. It also generates hydroxyl radicals by reaction with H_2O_2. Myeloperoxidase, found in the primary granules of neutrophils, catalyses the formation of the strong microbicidal agent hypochlorous acid from Cl^- and H_2O_2. The hypochlorous acid so formed reacts with amines to form chloramines.

Non-O_2-dependent microbicidal mechanisms include a reduction of pH within phagocytic vacuoles (phagosomes) and the release into phagosomes of (i) lysozyme (found within azurophilic and specific granules), which causes swelling and rupture of bacteria; (ii) defensins (peptides) and bacterial permeability increasing protein (both found in primary granules) that damage and make leaky the membranes of microorganisms; and (iii) the iron-binding protein lactoferrin, which may prevent ingested bacteria from taking up iron.

Lymphocytes

Between 65% and 80% of peripheral blood lymphocytes are T cells, 10–30% are B cells and 2–10% are non-T and non-B cells (null cells). Both B and T cells are formed with specific antigen-recognizing molecules on their cell surface which determine that each cell recognizes a specific antigenic determinant. The antigen-recognizing molecules for B and T cells are, respectively, immunoglobulin and the T-cell receptor (TCR) molecule. The cells are triggered into proliferation when they react with the specific antigen in the presence of appropriate accessory cells; their progeny develop into effector cells or memory cells.

The effector T-lymphocytes include helper cells (CD4+ cells), which promote the function of B cells and are required for the maturation of other types of T cell, and suppressor–cytotoxic cells (CD8+ cells), which inhibit the function of other lymphocytes and are cytotoxic towards foreign and virus-infected cells. The ratio of helper to suppressor cells is 1.5–2.5:1. Thus, the functions of the T cells include:

1 Mediation of cellular immunity against viruses, fungi and low-grade intracellular pathogens such as mycobacteria.
2 Participation in delayed hypersensitivity reactions, tumour rejection and graft rejection.
3 Interaction with B cells in producing antibodies against certain antigens.
4 Suppression of B-cell function.

Activated T cells also produce interleukin-5 (IL-5, eosinophil colony-stimulating factor) which is involved in the regulation of eosinophil granulocytopoiesis and IL-3, one of the multilineage haemopoietic growth factors. (This explains the excessive eosinophil production in some T-cell lymphomas.) They also produce other haemopoietic growth factors (IL-6, granulocyte–macrophage colony-stimulating factor (GM-CSF), granulocyte colony-stimulating factor (G-CSF), macrophage colony-stimulating factor (M-CSF)) (p. 15).

The percentages of B cells that express IgM, IgD, IgG and IgA molecules on their surface are, respectively, 40%, 30%, 30% and 10%. Many B cells have both IgM and IgD on their surface but others usually have only IgG or IgA. A single B cell expresses immunoglobulins of only one light chain type, and there are twice as many cells with κ light chains as there are with λ light chains. B cells that are activated by reaction with a specific antigen develop into antibody-secreting plasma cells or into B memory cells. Most of the antibodies formed during a primary antibody response consist of IgM, and almost all of the antibodies formed during a secondary antibody response (which results from the activation of B memory cells) consist of IgG.

The null cells are now known as natural killer (NK) cells. These cells lyse antibody-coated target cells and are therefore also called antibody-dependent cytotoxic cells (ADCC). The NK cells also kill tumour cells and virus-infected cells in the absence of antibody.

Further information on B cells, T cells and NK cells is provided in Chapter 7.

Haemopoiesis in the adult

In normal adults, haemopoiesis (production of blood cells) only occurs in the marrow contained within certain bones (p. 15).

General considerations and early events

Haemopoietic systems of adults are examples of steady-state cell renewal systems in which the rate of loss of mature cells (red cells, granulocytes, monocytes, lymphocytes and platelets) from the blood is balanced fairly precisely by the rate of release of newly formed cells into the blood. Mature cells are lost either because of ageing or during the performance of normal functions.

The formation of blood cells involves two processes:

1 Progressive development of structural and functional characteristics specific for a given cell type (cytodifferentiation or maturation).
2 Cell proliferation.

A schematic representation of haemopoiesis is shown in Fig. 1.7. The stem cells and progenitor cells are involved early in haemopoiesis; they cannot be recognized morphologically in marrow smears but can be studied by functional tests. In man, these cells (colony-forming units or CFU) have been identified and characterized on the basis of their ability to produce small colonies of one or more cell types when grown in semi-solid media containing appropriate haemopoietic growth factors. The most primitive haemopoietic cell is the pluripotent haemopoietic stem cell. This gives rise to two types of committed stem cell, namely multipotent myeloid stem cells and lymphoid stem cells. The essential characteristics of stem cells are:

1 An extensive capacity to maintain their own number by cell proliferation (self-renewal).
2 The capacity to mature into other cell types.

The lymphoid stem cells give rise to lymphocyte progenitor cells that eventually mature into all types of T and B lymphocytes and NK cells. The multipotent myeloid stem cells differentiate into various types of myeloid progenitor cell which eventually generate erythrocytes, neutrophils, eosinophils, basophils, monocytes, platelets, mast cells and osteoclasts. Unlike the stem cells, the lymphoid and myeloid progenitor cells have only a limited capacity for self-renewal.

The more immature myeloid progenitor cells are committed to two or three differentiation pathways. With increasing maturity, their differentiation potential becomes progressively limited, eventually to one pathway only. The unipotent progenitor cells committed to the production of erythrocytes, neutrophil granulocytes, eosinophil granulocytes, basophil granulocytes, monocytes/macrophages and megakaryocytes are, respectively, called CFU-E, CFU-G, CFU-eo, CFU-baso, CFU-M and CFU-mega. They mature into the earliest morphologically recognizable cells of the corresponding cell lineage (pronormoblasts, myeloblasts, monoblasts and megakaryoblasts).

Pluripotent haemopoietic stem cells account for about one per 10,000–100,000 nucleated marrow cells. They are also found in very small numbers in circulating blood so that stem cells used for marrow transplantation can be derived not only from bone marrow but also from peripheral blood. Haemopoietic progenitor cells are also found both in marrow and in blood. Despite their presence in blood, myeloid stem cells and progenitor cells normally develop into morphologically recognizable haemopoietic cells only within the microenvironment of the bone marrow.

In addition to haemopoietic stem cells, the marrow contains a more primitive cell type known as mesenchymal stem cells that gives rise to the pluripotent haemopoietic stem cells but may also differentiate under appropriate conditions *in vitro* and/or *in vivo* into a variety of non-haemopoietic cell types such as chondrocytes, osteoblasts, adipocytes, cardiac myocytes, hepatocytes and even neuronal cells.

Morphologically recognizable haemopoietic cells derived from myeloid stem cells

In every myeloid cell lineage other than that involved in platelet production, the early precursors

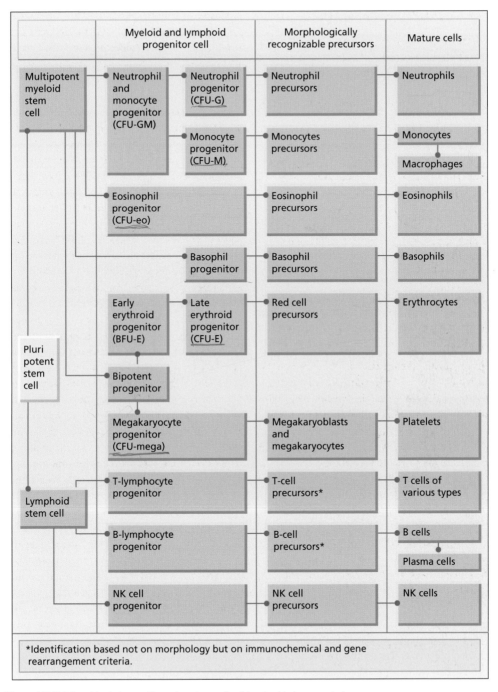

Figure 1.7 Relationships between the various types of cell involved in haemopoiesis.

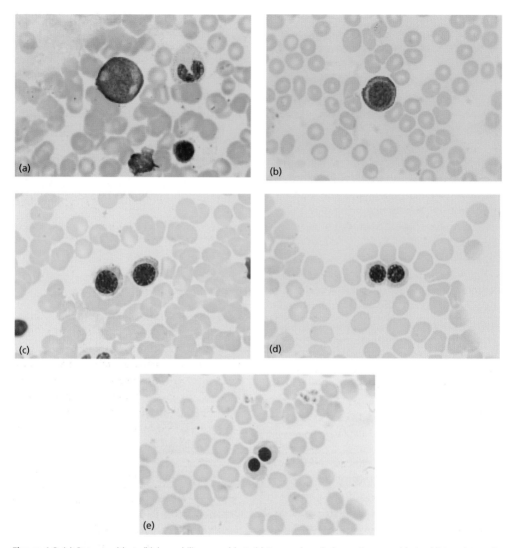

Figure 1.8 (a) Pronormoblast, (b) basophilic normoblast, (c) two early polychromatic normoblasts, (d) two late poly-chromatic normoblasts and (e) two more mature late polychromatic normoblasts. The granules of condensed chromatin in the basophilic normoblast are slightly coarser than in the pronormoblast. The nuclei of the late polychromatic normoblasts contain large masses of condensed chromatin.

that can be identified on morphological and cytochemical criteria are capable of both dividing and maturing. The late precursors do not divide but continue to mature. The proliferative activity during haemopoiesis serves as an amplifying mechanism and ensures that a large number of mature blood cells are derived from a single cell that becomes committed to any particular lineage.

Erythropoiesis

The pronormoblast is a large cell with a small quantity of agranular intensely basophilic cytoplasm (due to the presence of numerous ribosomes) and a large nucleus containing finely dispersed nuclear chromatin and nucleoli (Fig. 1.8(a)). The successive stages through which a pronormoblast develops into erythrocytes are termed basophilic normoblasts (Fig. 1.8(b)); early and late polychromatic normoblasts (Fig. 1.8(c)–(e)); marrow reticulocytes and blood reticulocytes. Pronormoblasts, basophilic normoblasts and early polychromatic normoblasts undergo cell division and the late polychromatic normoblasts do not. Nucleated cell classes of increasing maturity show: (i) a progressive reduction in cell and nuclear size; (ii) a progressive increase in the quantity of condensed nuclear chromatin; (iii) a progressive increase in the ratio of cytoplasmic volume to nuclear volume; and (iv) a progressive increase in Hb (which stains pink) and a progressive decrease in ribosomal RNA (which stains blue), resulting in polychromasia (grey–pink colour). The late polychromatic normoblast extrudes its nucleus and becomes a marrow reticulocyte. The marrow reticulocytes enter the blood stream and circulate for 1–2 days before becoming mature red cells.

In Romanowsky-stained marrow and blood smears, reticulocytes appear as rounded, faintly polychromatic cells whose diameters are slightly larger than those of mature red cells. When living polychromatic red cells are incubated with brilliant cresyl blue (supravital staining), the ribosomes form a basophilic precipitate of granules or filaments, or both; in the most immature of these cells the precipitated RNA appears as a basophilic reticulum (hence the term 'reticulocyte') (Fig. 1.9). Mature red cells lack ribosomes.

On the basis of their morphological features, nucleated red cell precursors (erythroblasts) found in normal marrow are called normoblasts and normal erythropoiesis is described as being normoblastic in type. The characteristic feature of normoblastic erythropoiesis is the presence of moderate quantities of condensed nuclear chromatin in early polychromatic erythroblasts. Even in healthy individuals, a few erythroblasts fail to develop normally and such cells are recognized and phagocytosed by bone marrow macrophages. This loss of potential erythrocytes due to the intramedullary destruction of red cell precursors is described as ineffective erythropoiesis. The extent of ineffective erythropoiesis in normal marrow is slight.

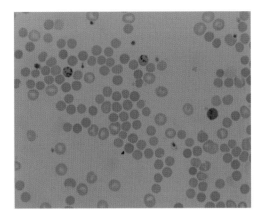

Figure 1.9 Reticulocytes in peripheral blood stained supravitally with brilliant cresyl blue. Note the reticulum of precipitated ribosomes.

Neutrophil granulocytopoiesis

The myeloblasts superficially resemble pronormoblasts except that their cytoplasm is less basophilic (Fig. 1.10(a)). The successive cytological classes through which a myeloblast matures into circulating neutrophil granulocytes are termed promyelocytes (Fig. 1.10(b)), neutrophil myelocytes (Fig. 1.10(c)), neutrophil metamyelocytes and neutrophil band cells (stab cells). During this maturation the following changes occur:

1 A progressive reduction of cytoplasmic basophilia and a progressive increase in the quantity of condensed chromatin after the promyelocyte stage.
2 The formation of coarse, purplish-red (azurophilic) cytoplasmic granules (primary granules) at the promyelocyte stage, which remain visible at the myelocyte stage but not later.
3 The formation of fine neutrophilic granules (specific granules) at the myelocyte and metamyelocyte stages.
4 Indentation of the nucleus which is moderate at the metamyelocyte stage (C-shaped nucleus) and more marked at the band cell stage (U-shaped, curved or coiled band-like nucleus).
5 A progressive segmentation of the U-shaped or band-like nucleus of the band cell leading to the formation of granulocytes with two to five nuclear lobes.

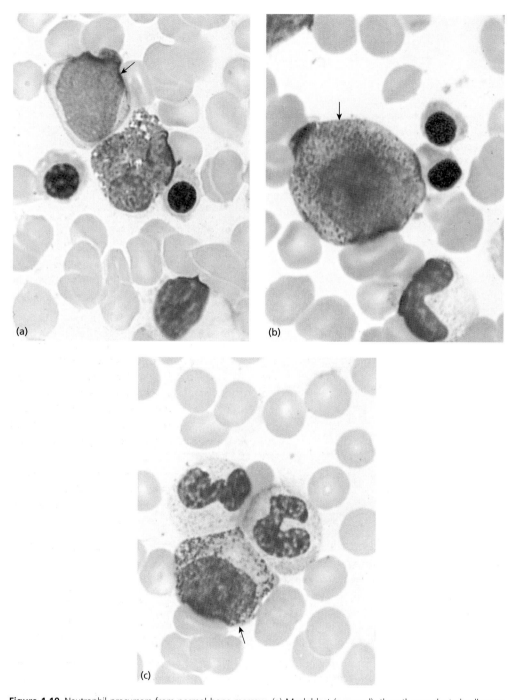

Figure 1.10 Neutrophil precursors from normal bone marrow. (a) Myeloblast (arrowed); the other nucleated cells near the myeloblast are an eosinophil granulocyte (centre) and two polychromatic erythroblasts. (b) Promyelocyte (arrowed); the other nucleated cells are two polychromatic erythroblasts and a neutrophil metamyelocyte. (c) Neutrophil myelocyte (arrowed); there are two neutrophil band cells adjacent to the myelocyte.

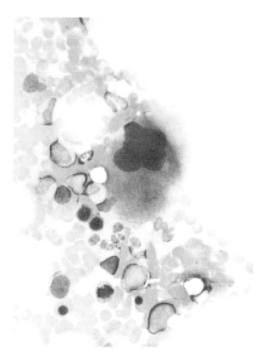

Figure 1.11 Mature megakaryocyte (centre). This is a very large cell with a single lobulated nucleus. Compare the size of the megakaryocyte with that of the other nucleated marrow cells in this figure.

Cell division occurs in myeloblasts, promyelocytes and myelocytes but not normally in metamyelocytes and band cells.

Megakaryocytopoiesis

During megakaryocytopoiesis, there is replication of DNA without nuclear or cell division which leads to the generation of very large uninucleate cells with DNA contents between 8c and 64c (other haemopoietic cells have DNA contents between 2c and 4c; 1c is the DNA content of a germ cell). There is a rough correlation between the DNA content of a megakaryocyte nucleus and both its size and extent of lobulation. A mature megakaryocyte is illustrated in Fig. 1.11. Large numbers of platelets are formed from the cytoplasm of each mature megakaryocyte; these are rapidly discharged directly into the marrow

sinusoids. The residual 'bare' megakaryocyte nucleus is phagocytosed by macrophages.

Monocytopoiesis

The cell classes belonging to the monocyte–macrophage lineage (the mononuclear phagocyte system) are, in increasing order of maturity: monoblasts, promonocytes, marrow monocytes, blood monocytes and tissue macrophages.

Lymphocytopoiesis

The lymphoid stem cell in the bone marrow generates B-cell progenitors within that tissue. The B-cell progenitors undergo maturation into B cells in the microenvironment of the marrow and then travel via the blood into the B-cell zones of peripheral lymphoid tissue (follicles and medulla of lymph nodes and splenic follicles).

Either the lymphoid stem cells or primitive T-cell progenitors derived from them migrate from the marrow, via the blood, into the thymus where maturation into T cells takes place; those T cells that recognize self are deleted. The T cells later migrate to the T-cell zones of peripheral lymphoid organs (paracortical areas and medulla of lymph nodes and periarteriolar lymphoid sheaths of the spleen).

The terms used to describe cells at various stages of B-lymphocyte differentiation in the bone marrow and T-lymphocyte differentiation in the thymus are as follows:

Pre-pre-B cell → pre-B cell → immature B cell →
mature B cell

Pre-T cell (thymic lymphoblast) → early thymocyte (large cortical thymocyte) → intermediate thymocyte (small cortical thymocyte) → late thymocyte (medullary thymocyte) → mature T cell

All these stages have the morphological features of either lymphoblasts or lymphocytes. The identification of different lymphocyte precursors is therefore based not on morphology but on various properties like reactivity with certain monoclonal antibodies, immunoglobulin gene rearrangement status, presence of immunoglobulin

Table 1.4 The sequence of events during B-cell differentiation.

Characteristic	Pre-pre-B cell	Pre-B cell	Immature B cell	Mature B cell	Plasma cell
Heavy-chain genes rearranged	+	+	+	+	+
Light-chain genes rearranged	−/+	+	+	+	+
Terminal deoxynucleotidyl-transferase	+	+/−	−	−	−
Cytoplasmic μ-chains expressed	−	+	−	−	−
Surface IgM (but not IgD) expressed	−	−	+	−	−
Surface IgM and IgD expressed	−	−	−	+	−
Cytoplasmic Ig expressed	−	−	−	−	+
cALLA (CD10)	+	+	−	−	−
CD19 and CD20	+	+	+	+	+

Note: cALLA — common acute lymphoblastic leukaemia antigen.

Table 1.5 The sequence of events during T-cell differentiation.

Characteristic	Pre-T cell	Early thymocyte	Intermediate thymocyte	Late thymocyte	Mature T cell
CD7	+	+	+	+	+
Terminal deoxynucleotidyl-transferase	−/+	+	+	−	−
TCR γ genes rearranged/deleted	−	+	+	+	+
TCR β genes rearranged	−	−	+	+	+
TCR α genes rearranged	−	−	−/+	+	+
CD2	−	+	+	+	+
CD3	−	+	+	+	+
CD4 and CD8	−	−	−/+	−	−
CD4 or CD8	−	−	−	+	+

Note: TCR — T-cell receptor.

on the surface membrane, presence of μ-chains or immunoglobulin within the cytoplasm, terminal deoxynucleotidyl-transferase (TdT) activity and TCR gene rearrangement status (Tables 1.4 and 1.5) (also see Chapter 7).

Regulation of haemopoiesis

The regulation of haemopoietic cells, including haemopoietic stem cells and progenitor cells, depends on intimate contact with one or more types of bone marrow stromal cell (macrophages, endothelial cells, fibroblasts, adipocytes and osteoblasts) and with stromal-cell-derived extracellular matrix components. The stromal cells (and also some T-lymphocytes) influence the proliferation and maturation of the haemopoietic stem cells and progenitor cells by producing: (i) a number of membrane-bound, matrix-bound and soluble haemopoietic growth factors; and (ii) inhibitory cytokines (e.g. transforming growth factor-β, tumour necrosis factor (TNF), and interferons). Haemopoietic growth factors are also produced by the liver (thrombopoietin (TPO) and <10% of the erythropoietin) and kidneys (most of the eythropoietin). One of the important growth factors acting on stem cells is called stem-cell factor (SCF, kit ligand or Steel factor). Growth factors influencing early progenitor cells include SCF, IL-3, TPO and GM-CSF. Those acting on the lineage-committed bipotent or unipotent progenitor cells include G-CSF, M-CSF, IL-5 (influencing CFU-eo), TPO (influencing CFU-mega) and erythropoietin. Haemopoietic growth factors react with specific receptors on the cell membrane of target cells and mediate their effects on survival, proliferation and differentiation via second messengers. In their absence, the target cell undergoes programmed cell death (apoptosis). All the haemopoietic growth factors are glycoproteins and some (erythropoietin, GM-CSF, G-CSF) have been genetically engineered and are available as therapeutic agents. Growth factors such as G-CSF and GM-CSF not only influence haemopoiesis but also enhance the function of the mature cells.

The details of the steady-state regulation of blood cells other than red cells are still not entirely clear. The rate of erythropoiesis is primarily regulated by the hormone erythropoietin, which is secreted mainly by the kidneys, probably by peritubular cells. The production of erythropoietin is stimulated when the supply of oxygen to renal tissue falls (e.g. when the red cell count falls). Erythropoietin increases red cell production mainly by stimulating the rate of conversion of CFU-E to pronormoblasts. It also shortens the total time taken for a pronormoblast to mature into marrow reticulocytes and for the latter to be released into the circulation.

Intrauterine haemopoiesis and postnatal changes

The production of blood cells begins in the yolk sac of the 14- to 19-day human embryo. The fetal liver becomes the main site of haemopoiesis in the second trimester of pregnancy and the fetal bone marrow in the third trimester. The majority of the haemopoietic cells in the yolk sac and fetal liver are erythroblasts. The embryonic Hbs, Gower 1 ($\zeta_2\varepsilon_2$), Gower 2 ($\alpha_2\varepsilon_2$) and Portland 1 ($\zeta_2\gamma_2$), are synthesized by erythroblasts in the yolk sac, fetal Hb (HbF, $\alpha_2\gamma_2$) by erythroblasts in the fetal liver, and both HbF and HbA ($\alpha_2\beta_2$) by those in the fetal bone marrow. The main site of granulocytopoietic activity in intrauterine life is the fetal bone marrow.

After birth, the marrow is the sole site of haemopoiesis in healthy individuals. During the first 4 years of life, nearly all the marrow cavities contain red haemopoietic marrow with very few fat cells. Thereafter, increasing numbers of fat cells appear in certain marrow cavities. By the age of 25 years, the only sites of active haemopoiesis are the skull bones, ribs, sternum, scapulae, clavicles, vertebrae, pelvis, the upper half of the sacrum, and the proximal ends of the shafts of the femur and humerus. All the remaining marrow cavities contain yellow fatty marrow. Even at sites of active haemopoiesis, about half the volume of the marrow normally consists of fat cells.

In a number of diseases (e.g. chronic haemolytic anaemias, megaloblastic anaemias and some leukaemias) there may be: (i) a partial or complete replacement of fat cells by haemopoietic cells in marrow cavities normally supporting haemopoiesis; (ii) the extension of haemopoietic marrow into marrow cavities normally containing non-haemopoietic fatty marrow (e.g. in long bones); and (iii) the appearance of foci of haemopoietic tissue in the liver and spleen (extramedullary haemopoiesis).

Chapter 2

Anaemia and Polycythaemia: General Considerations

Learning objectives

- To know how the symptoms and signs of anaemia and polycythaemia are caused.
- To understand the mechanisms of production of anaemia.
- To understand the morphological classification and diagnostic approaches to anaemia.
- To know the causes of true and apparent polycythaemia.

Table 2.1 Reference ranges for Hb values.

	Hb concentration (g/dL)
Cord blood	13.5–20.5
First day of life	15.0–23.5
Children, 6 months–6 years	11.0–14.5
Children, 6–14 years	12.0–15.5
Adult males	13.0–17.0
Adult females (non-pregnant)	12.0–15.5
Pregnant females	11.0–14.0

Anaemia

Anaemia is said to be present when the haemoglobin (Hb) concentration is below the reference range (reference interval) for the age and sex of an individual. Reference ranges are derived from the statistical analysis of data from a sample of reference individuals (i.e. individuals selected on the basis of defined criteria). Reference ranges for Hb concentration are given in Table 2.1. These may be determined from a representative sample of healthy persons in whom the presence of iron deficiency has been excluded by specific laboratory investigations or by the prior administration of iron. In populations with a high prevalence of α- and β-thalassaemia genes, heterozygosity for thalassaemia may also have to be excluded. The average Hb level is 17.0 g/dL at birth and rises to 19.5 g/dL after 24 h. Hb levels in children between 6 months and 6 years tend to be lower than in adults. The higher Hb levels in adult males than in adult non-pregnant females are largely due to the effects of higher androgen levels in males; the Hb levels of males fall after the age of 70 years. Hb levels are increased by residence at high altitude. Hb levels decrease during normal pregnancy, reaching their lowest value at about 32 weeks; the average fall is 1.5–2.0 g/dL. The drop in Hb concentration occurs despite an average increase in red cell mass of 300 mL, and results from an average increase in the plasma volume of about 1 L. The Hb level may drop by 6–8% after about half an hour of bed rest.

Although reference ranges are invaluable in the assessment of a patient, it must be realized that they do have some limitations. Thus, since reference

Lecture Notes: Haematology, by NC Hughes-Jones, SN Wickramsinghe, CSR Hatton © 2008 Blackwell Publishing, ISBN: 9781405180504

ranges represent 95% reference limits determined on a healthy population, it would be expected that 2.5% of healthy individuals have Hb values below and 2.5% above the reference range. Therefore, not all individuals with Hb levels slightly outside the reference range would necessarily have some haematological problem. Furthermore, as the difference between the upper and lower limits of the reference range is more than 3.0 g/dL, an individual's Hb level may remain within the reference range even though it has fallen substantially due to some illness. In other words, a 'normal' Hb concentration does not necessarily exclude impairment of erythropoiesis. It also does not exclude a moderate reduction in red cell lifespan as the healthy bone marrow has a considerable physiological reserve and can increase the rate of effective erythropoiesis to 6–8 times the basal rate. In patients with both anaemia and a decrease in the plasma volume secondary to dehydration, the Hb level may be spuriously high.

In healthy individuals, there are strong correlations between the Hb, red cell count and packed cell volume (PCV). The reference ranges for the red cell count in adult males and females are, respectively, 4.4–5.8 and 4.1–5.2 $\times$ 10^{12}/L. The reference ranges for the PCV in adult males and females are 0.40–0.51 and 0.36–0.48 respectively.

Adaptive responses to anaemia

An important compensatory mechanism in anaemia consists of an increased production of 2,3-diphosphoglycerate (2,3-DPG) by red cells. This causes a reduction in the O_2 affinity of Hb (a shift of the O_2 dissociation curve to the right) and, consequently, an increased release of O_2 at the tissues (p. 1). When the Hb falls below 7–8 g/dL, adaptive changes also occur in the cardiovascular system: these include an increase of cardiac output at rest mainly by an increase in stroke volume, but also by an increase in heart rate.

Symptoms and signs of anaemia

Anaemia is a manifestation of disease, not a final diagnosis. The symptoms found in an anaemic patient may be caused by the underlying disease or by the anaemia itself. When anaemia develops slowly in children and young adults, the symptoms referable to the anaemia are mild until the Hb falls below 7–8 g/dL. Significant symptoms develop at higher Hb levels in rapidly developing anaemias and in older patients with impaired cardiovascular reserves. Older patients are also more likely to develop cardiac and cerebral symptoms than younger ones, due to associated degenerative vascular disease.

The two mechanisms underlying the many symptoms and signs of anaemia are:

1 Decreased tissue oxygenation causing widespread organ dysfunction.
2 Adaptive changes, particularly in the cardiovascular system.

Symptoms include lassitude, easy fatiguability, dyspnoea on exertion, palpitation, angina and intermittent claudication (in older patients with degenerative arterial disease), headache, vertigo, light-headedness, visual disturbances, drowsiness, anorexia, nausea, bowel disturbances, menstrual disturbances and loss of libido. Physical signs include pallor, tachycardia, wide pulse pressure with capillary pulsation, haemic murmurs, signs of congestive cardiac failure, and haemorrhages and occasional exudates in the retina. Severe anaemia may also cause slight proteinuria, mild impairment of renal function and low-grade fever.

Mechanisms of anaemia

In healthy adults, there is a steady-state equilibrium between the rate of release of new red cells from the bone marrow into the circulation and the rate of removal of senescent red cells from the circulation by macrophages. The various mechanisms which may lead to anaemia are shown in Table 2.2. More than one of these mechanisms operate simultaneously in most conditions, and mechanistic classifications of the anaemias have to be based on the mechanism of greatest pathophysiological importance. Impaired red cell formation may be due to insufficient erythropoiesis (reduced quantity of erythropoietic

Table 2.2 Various mechanisms leading to anaemia.

Blood loss
Decreased red cell lifespan (haemolytic anaemia)
Congenital defect (e.g. sickle-cell disease, hereditary spherocytosis)
Acquired defect (e.g. malaria, some drugs)
Impairment of red cell formation
Insufficient erythropoiesis
Ineffective erythropoiesis
Pooling and destruction of red cells in an enlarged spleen
Increased plasma volume (splenomegaly, pregnancy)

tissue) or to ineffective erythropoiesis (a high death rate affecting the red cell precursors within the marrow).

The absolute reticulocyte count (i.e., the number of reticulocytes per litre of blood) is a useful parameter with which anaemias due to increased red cell destruction can be distinguished from those due to impaired red cell production. This count is a relatively easily determined index of the rate of delivery of red cells into the circulation (i.e. of effective erythropoiesis). The absolute reticulocyte count (pp. 27 and 183) is increased in haemolytic anaemias as well as after acute blood loss and after treatment of iron, vitamin B_{12} or folate-deficient patients with the appropriate haematinic. Reticulocyte counts are low or normal when anaemia is due to impaired red cell production.

Blood loss

The loss of 500 mL of blood over a few minutes usually has negligible effects on the circulatory system: there is a slight fall in central venous pressure and no significant change in blood pressure or pulse rate. The rapid loss of 750 mL causes a substantial fall in central venous pressure, a fall in cardiac output and blood pressure and peripheral vasoconstriction. The acute loss of 1.5–2.0 L of blood causes marked circulatory disturbances: the subjects are cold, clammy and restless, and may become unconscious.

Immediately after an acute haemorrhage, the Hb level is normal. The acute reduction in blood

volume is corrected by a slow expansion of the plasma volume over the next 36–72 h. This results in the gradual development of a normochromic normocytic anaemia, with the lowest Hb values between 36 and 72 h. Other changes seen in the blood after acute haemorrhage include:

1 Reticulocytosis (with a peak at 7–10 days).
2 Moderate neutrophil leucocytosis and mild thrombocytosis lasting for several days.
3 The presence of metamyelocytes and occasional myelocytes in the blood film. Normoblasts may appear in the blood after severe haemorrhage.

Chronic blood loss eventually causes a hypochromic microcytic anaemia due to iron deficiency.

Other mechanisms

The anaemias resulting partly or wholly from a substantial reduction of red cell lifespan are discussed in Chapter 3. The diseases associated with impaired red cell formation are listed in Table 2.3. In chronic renal failure, anaemia is mainly caused by decreased erythropoietin production in the diseased kidneys and usually responds to parenteral therapy with recombinant human erythropoietin. Anaemia develops in endocrine deficiency syndromes because normal erythropoiesis, which is dependent on the erythroid lineage-specific hormone erythropoietin, is also influenced by some secretions of the endocrine glands, particularly androgens and thyroxine.

Morphological classification of anaemias

A useful method for classifying anaemias is based on the morphology of red cells in a stained blood smear. The main terms used in such a classification are normocytic, microcytic, macrocytic, normochromic and hypochromic. *Normocytes* are red cells with a normal diameter; *microcytes* and *macrocytes* are those with a reduced and increased diameter, respectively (Fig. 2.1(a)–(c)). *Normochromia* implies normal staining of the cell, with the central area of pallor occupying about a third of the cell diameter (Fig. 2.1(a)) and *hypochromia* indicates reduced staining, with an

Table 2.3 Causes of anaemia due to impaired red cell formation.

Deficiency of essential haematinics
Iron, folate, vitamin B_{12}, protein (see Chapters 4 and 5)

Chronic disorders (p. 58)
Infection, renal disease, liver disease, collagen disease

Marrow infiltration
Carcinoma, myeloma, leukaemia, lymphoma, myelofibrosis, lysosomal storage diseases (e.g. Gaucher's disease), marble bone disease

Endocrine deficiency
Hypofunction of the thyroid (p. 77), testes or anterior lobe of the pituitary gland

Myelotoxic agents, aplastic anaemia and pure red cell aplasia

Miscellaneous
Vitamin B_{12}-independent and folate-independent megaloblastic anaemias, β-thalassaemia syndromes, myelodysplastic syndromes (including primary acquired sideroblastic anaemia), congenital dyserythropoietic anaemias, malaria

---

increase in the central area of pallor (Fig. 2.1(b)). Today, morphological classification is based not only on morphological criteria but also on mean cell volumes (MCV) determined by automated blood-counting machines. It must be appreciated, however, that when blood contains only a small proportion of microcytes or macrocytes, the MCV is within the normal range. The three morphological types of anaemia and examples of conditions causing them are given in Table 2.4. The normal values for the MCV and other red cell indices in adults are given in Table 2.5.

There are a number of morphological abnormalities of red cells other than those mentioned above which may be seen on a stained blood film in a patient with anaemia; some of these are mentioned below.

Anisocytosis and poikilocytosis

An increased degree of variation in cell diameter (anisocytosis) or cell shape (poikilocytosis) may be seen in many conditions associated with disturbed erythropoiesis. They are not specific for any disease.

Target cells

These are abnormal red cells which have a well-stained area in their middle and periphery and a pale area in between (Fig. 2.1(d) and (e)); this appearance results from the presence of excess cell membrane relative to the volume of the cytoplasm. Target cells are found in thalassaemia syndromes, iron deficiency, sickle-cell anaemia, heterozygotes and homozygotes for HbC, homozygotes for HbE, liver disease, obstructive jaundice, hyposplenism and splenectomized individuals.

Spherocytes or microspherocytes

In several different types of haemolytic anaemia, some red cells lose their biconcave shape and become more or less spherical. In blood films, they appear as deeply stained cells that have lost their central area of pallor and that have smaller diameters than normal cells (Fig. 2.1(d)). Spherocytes have a reduced surface/volume ratio and usually result from:

1 An inherited abnormality of the red cell membrane cytoskeleton (hereditary spherocytosis).
2 An acquired abnormality of the red cell membrane (e.g. damage by clostridial toxin, or by heat, as in patients with burns).
3 Ingestion of part of an antibody-coated red cell by a macrophage, as in autoimmune haemolytic anaemias with warm-reactive antibodies.
4 Loss of fragments from circulating red cells by their mechanical interaction with fibrin strands or diseased vessel walls, as in microangiopathic haemolytic anaemia.

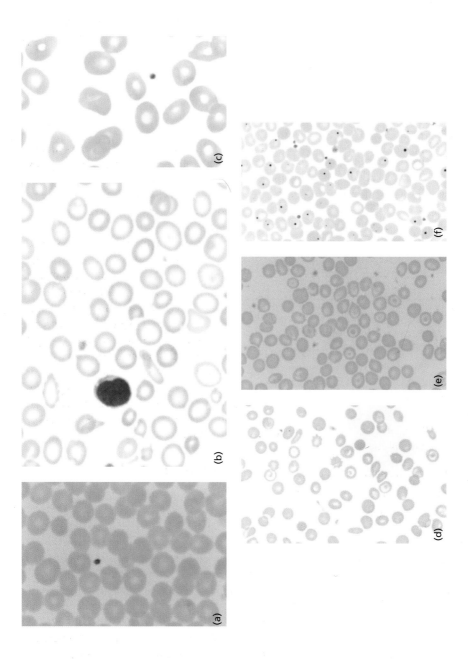

Figure 2.1 Normal and abnormal red cells: (a) Normochromic, normocytic cells. (b) Hypochromic, microcytic cells. (c) Oval macrocytes and a poikilocyte. (d) Target cells, spherocytes and acanthocytes in a blood film from a splenectomized patient. Acanthocytes are red cells with up to about 10 spicules of varying length irregularly distributed over their surface. They are found not only postsplenectomy but also in other conditions such as hypothyroidism and advanced alcohol-related cirrhosis of the liver. (e) Target cells from a patient with obstructive jaundice; (f) Howell–Jolly bodies within red cells. Figures (a)–(c) are at similar magnification; (d)–(f) are at a lower magnification.

Table 2.4 Morphological classification of anaemia.

Type	MCV	Causes
Microcytic and hypochromic, or microcytic*	Low	Iron deficiency, thalassaemia syndromes, some cases of anaemia of chronic disorders
Normocytic and normochromic	Normal	Acute blood loss, some cases of anaemia of chronic disorders, chronic renal failure, some haemolytic anaemias, leucoerythroblastic anaemias
Macrocytic	High	Alcoholism, folate deficiency, vitamin B_{12} deficiency (see Chapter 6 for other causes)

Notes: MCV — mean cell volume.

* Microcytic red cells do not always appear hypochromic on a blood film.

Table 2.5 Reference ranges for red cell indices in adults.

Index	Normal range
Mean cell volume* (MCV)	82–99 fL
Mean cell Hb (MCH)	27–33 pg
Mean cell Hb concentration (MCHC)	32–36 g/dL

Note: * Lower limit may be as low as 70–74 fL between 1 and 8 years of age, in the absence of iron deficiency.

Howell–Jolly bodies

These small, rounded intraerythrocytic inclusions consist of nuclear material. They are found in circulating red cells following splenectomy or in patients with hyposplenism. Howell–Jolly bodies (Fig. 2.1(f)) are normally present in some red cells when they leave the marrow but are rapidly removed by the spleen, possibly during the first passage of the inclusion containing cells through that organ. Consequently, they are not found in blood films of individuals with a functioning spleen. In megaloblastic anaemias the formation of Howell–Jolly bodies within the erythroblasts in the marrow is greatly increased, and when megaloblastic haemopoiesis is associated with splenectomy or hyposplenism, the peripheral blood contains very large numbers of red cells with these inclusions.

Polycythaemia (erythrocytosis)

The term 'polycythaemia' is usually applied when the PCV is repeatedly greater than 0.51 in adult males and 0.48 in adult females in peripheral blood samples taken without venous occlusion. The increase in PCV is associated with a high Hb level and a high red cell count. Polycythaemia may result either from an increase in the total volume of red cells in the circulation (true polycythaemia) or from a decrease in the total plasma volume (apparent or relative polycythaemia). Thus, measurements of total red cell volume (using ^{51}Cr- or ^{99m}Tc-labelled red cells) and plasma volume (using ^{125}I-albumin) are often required in the investigation of patients. The total red cell volume (red cell mass) is expressed as a percentage of the value predicted for the gender, height and weight of the individual being studied. A patient is considered to have true polycythaemia when the measured red cell mass exceeds the predicted value by more than 25%. The disorders associated with true and apparent polycythaemia are given in Table 2.6.

True polycythaemia

An important cause of true polycythaemia, namely polycythaemia vera, is discussed on p. 130. In most of the conditions listed as causing true polycythaemia due to inappropriate erythropoietin production in Table 2.6, the increased amounts of erythropoietin are either secreted by tumour cells or by compressed and hypoxic normal renal tissue surrounding renal cysts or tumours. Occasionally, there may be increased production of erythropoietin in the absence of generalized hypoxia due to an impairment of renal blood flow causing selective renal hypoxia. From the many causes of secondary polycythaemia shown, it is evident that diagnosis

Table 2.6 Causes of true and apparent polycythaemia.

Classification of polycythaemia	
True polycythaemia (increased red cell mass)	**Apparent polycythaemia (relative polycythaemia) (normal red cell mass)**
PRIMARY*	*Dehydration or plasma loss*
Polycythaemia vera	Vomiting
	Diarrhoea
SECONDARY	Inadequate fluid intake
Due to generalized tissue hypoxia causing appropriately increased erythropoietin production	Burns
High altitude, cyanotic heart disease, chronic hypoxic pulmonary disease, alveolar hypoventilation due to gross obesity, heavy smoking (formation of carboxyhaemoglobin), abnormal Hbs with high O_2 affinity (e.g., Hb Chesapeake)	*Chronic apparent polycythaemia* (also called stress polycythaemia or Gaisböck's syndrome) Associated with obesity, hypertension, diuretic therapy, heavy smoking and high alcohol intake
Due to inappropriately increased erythropoietin production	
Kidney disease (carcinoma, cysts, hydronephrosis), renal transplantation, hepatocellular carcinoma, cerebellar haemangioblastoma, massive uterine fibromyomatomas	
IDIOPATHIC	
Idiopathic erythrocytosis	

Note: *Abnormality originates in the marrow.

of the cause of a true polycythaemia may require a number of investigations, such as the measurement of the O_2 saturation of arterial blood, Hb electrophoresis (which detects two-thirds of the abnormal Hbs with a high O_2 affinity), determination of Hb–O_2 dissociation curves, abdominal ultrasound imaging, intravenous pyelography and measurement of serum erythropoietin levels.

True polycythaemia due to any cause is accompanied by an increase in whole blood viscosity. When symptoms are present, they generally result from a decrease in blood flow through the limbs, heart and brain as a consequence of the increased viscosity. Symptoms include headache, dizziness, fainting, fatigue, myalgia, muscle weakness, visual disturbances, confusion, somnolence that may progress to stupor or coma, paraesthesiae, breathlessness and chest pain. In polycythaemia vera, there is a high incidence of vaso-occlusive episodes related partly to the

hyperviscosity and partly to a high platelet count. The risk of vaso-occlusive episodes in secondary polycythaemia has not yet been adequately documented and may be less than in polycythaemia vera. However, thrombotic episodes are encountered in patients with polycythaemia secondary to cyanotic congenital heart disease and occasionally in patients with high-affinity Hbs.

Whereas venesection has a clear role in the management of polycythaemia vera (p. 130), its role in the management of secondary polycythaemia is less clear-cut since, in this situation, the increased red cell mass is an adaptation to lowered arterial O_2 saturation. In considering the possible value of venesection, the advantage of the decreased viscosity and consequent increased tissue perfusion has to be balanced against the disadvantage from a decreased O_2-carrying capacity. In cyanotic congenital heart disease, those patients with symptoms attributable to hyperviscosity

(Table 2.7) should have isovolaemic venesection bringing their PCV down to about 0.55. Repeated venesections should not be performed merely because the PCV is very high as this results in the development of microcytosis due to iron deficiency, increased viscosity and possibly increased risk of vasoocclusive events. Patients with polycythaemia secondary to hypoxic pulmonary disease should be considered for long-term oxygen therapy. In those with hyperviscosity symptoms or a PCV > 0.56 venesection down to a PCV of 0.50–0.52 (but not lower) has been shown in some studies to improve exercise tolerance, cardiac function and cerebral blood flow.

Apparent polycythaemia

This is commonly found as a temporary phenomenon when fluid balance is disturbed, with fluid loss exceeding fluid intake (Table 2.6).

Chronic apparent polycythaemia (spurious or stress polycythaemia) is a condition which has been reported especially in middle-aged men who are often anxious, hypertensive and obese. It is frequently associated with excessive alcohol consumption, low-dose diuretic therapy and smoking and may not be a single clinical entity. The PCV is raised but the red cell mass is normal. This group includes

Table 2.7 Symptoms of hyperviscosity in polycythaemic cyanotic patients.

Headache
Faintness and dizziness
Blurred vision, amaurosis fugax
Fatigue
Myalgia, muscle weakness
Paraesthesiae
Depressed mental function, sense of distance
Chest and abdominal pain

some normal individuals with a red cell mass at the upper limit of normal and a plasma volume at the lower limit of normal. In about 20% of cases, the plasma volume is reduced, sometimes to a marked degree.

Management consists of a reduction or cessation of alcohol intake and smoking, control of hypertension without the use of thiazide diuretics, and weight loss. If there is a recent history of thrombosis or there are risk factors for thrombosis with a PCV consistently above 0.54, venesection to a PCV of 0.45 should be considered based on the possibility that the prevalence of thromboembolic disorders may be as high as in polycythemia vera.

Chapter 3

Haemolytic Anaemias

Learning objectives

- To know the tests for recognizing:
  - that red cells are being destroyed at an excessive rate and
  - that the marrow is producing cells at a rate in excess of normal.
- To know the division of haemolytic anaemias into congenital and acquired, and to know the aetiological factors in each division.
- To understand the mode of inheritance, biochemical basis and clinical and laboratory features of hereditary spherocytosis (HS).
- To understand the role of glucose-6-phosphate dehydrogenase (G6PD) in glucose metabolism and the pathogenesis and clinical characteristics of the haemolytic syndromes that may be associated with a deficiency of this enzyme.
- To understand the ways in which abnormalities in the structure and rate of synthesis of globin chains cause clinical and haematological abnormalities.
- To know the clinical and laboratory manifestations of sickle-cell anaemia and the common thalassaemia syndromes, and to have a general understanding of the ethnic groups in which such abnormalities are likely to occur.
- To understand the role of autoantibodies in the production of haemolytic anaemias and to know the types of disease with which they are associated.
- To know some of the causes of non-immune acquired haemolytic anaemias.

Lecture Notes: Haematology, by NC Hughes-Jones, SN Wickramsinghe, CSR Hatton © 2008 Blackwell Publishing, ISBN: 9781405180504

The haemolytic anaemias are a group of diseases in which red cell lifespan is shortened. It should be noted that a patient with a diminished red cell lifespan is not always anaemic. When the rate of red cell destruction is increased, red cell production in the marrow is stimulated through the erythropoietin mechanism in an attempt to maintain the haemoglobin (Hb) concentration at the normal level. In the majority of haemolytic anaemias, the marrow responds optimally to this stimulus and increases the red cell output up to a maximum of 6–8 times normal. Thus, when patients have only a moderately reduced red cell lifespan, say 20–30 days instead of the normal 120 days, they increase the rate of red cell production sufficiently to maintain the Hb concentration within normal limits, provided that their Hb does not give up O_2 more readily than normal and their bone marrow is healthy. Such individuals are described as having a compensated haemolytic state rather than a haemolytic anaemia. On the other hand, a lifespan of 5–10 days, irrespective of its cause, is always associated with anaemia.

A suboptimal marrow response is seen when there is a lack of iron, vitamin B_{12} or folic acid; when the red cell precursors are damaged (sometimes by the agent causing the haemolysis); when the marrow is infiltrated by malignant cells (e.g. in chronic lymphocytic leukaemia complicated by an autoimmune haemolytic anaemia (AIHA)); and when there is increased ineffective erythropoiesis such as in homozygous β-thalassaemia.

In the majority of haemolytic anaemias, the macrophages in the spleen, liver and bone marrow remove the abnormal red cells from the circulation by phagocytosis (extravascular haemolysis). In a minority, the red cells rupture and release their Hb intravascularly (intravascular haemolysis).

The most commonly encountered haemolytic anaemias/states include hereditary spherocytosis (HS), hereditary elliptocytosis, glucose-6-phosphate dehydrogenase (G6PD) deficiency, sickle-cell anaemia, thalassaemia and the acquired haemolytic anaemias.

Evidence of haemolysis

Two categories of laboratory evidence can be looked for in a patient suspected of suffering from a haemolytic state. These are: (i) evidence of increased red cell destruction and (ii) evidence of a compensatory increase in erythropoietic activity.

Laboratory evidence of increased red cell destruction

The various types of evidence in this category are summarized in Table 3.1.

Biochemical consequences of extravascular haemolysis

The simplest method of obtaining evidence of increased red cell destruction is by estimating the amount of unconjugated bilirubin in plasma. When the red cell is destroyed within macrophages, the haem is converted into bilirubin with the release of carbon monoxide. Unconjugated bilirubin is insoluble in water and hence is transported to the liver attached to albumin. In the liver it is converted into the soluble glucuronide and excreted. The healthy liver is capable of handling more bilirubin than is normally produced and is able to increase its bilirubin-handling capacity further in haemolytic states. However,

Table 3.1 Laboratory findings indicative of increased red cell destruction.

Increased destruction
Biochemical consequences of extravascular haemolysis
Hyperbilirubinaemia (unconjugated)
Reduced serum haptoglobin
Biochemical consequences of intravascular haemolysis
Reduced serum haptoglobin
Haemoglobinaemia
Haemoglobinuria
Haemosiderinuria
Methaemalbuminaemia*
Morphological evidence of damage to red cells
Microspherocytes, red cell fragments, sickle cells
Reduced red cell lifespan

Note: * Now rarely used in investigating a patient.

there is an upper limit for the rate of glucuronide formation by the liver and when the supply of bilirubin exceeds this rate, the unconjugated bilirubin concentration in the plasma rises. Bilirubin concentration therefore does not rise above the normal range when there is only a moderate increase in the rate of destruction of red cells. It begins to rise when the lifespan is shortened to about 50 days or less. A rise in plasma bilirubin concentration is only significant in the diagnosis of a haemolytic process if liver function is entirely normal.

Biochemical consequences of intravascular haemolysis

The Hb released from intravascular lysis of red cells binds to the specific Hb-binding protein in the plasma, namely haptoglobin. Since the Hb–haptoglobin complexes are rapidly taken up by hepatocytes, intravascular haemolysis leads to a reduction in haptoglobin levels. Haptoglobins are also reduced in extravascular haemolysis, due to the escape of some Hb from the macrophages when they phagocytose damaged red cells.

When the quantity of Hb released during intravascular haemolysis exceeds the Hb binding

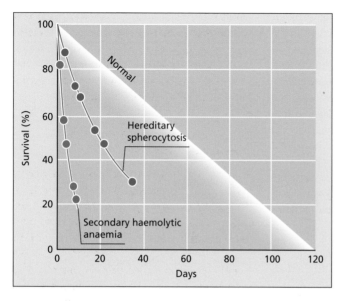

Figure 3.1 The survival of ^{51}Cr-labelled red cells (corrected for ^{51}Cr elution) in the circulation of a patient with HS (●), whose Hb concentration was 15.5 g/dL and mean red cell lifespan was 30 days; and in a patient with autoimmune haemolytic anaemia secondary to chronic lymphocytic leukaemia (●), whose Hb concentration was 5 g/dL and mean red cell lifespan was 5 days.

capacity of haptoglobin, free Hb is found in the plasma (haemoglobinaemia). Haem is released from the Hb and rapidly becomes oxidized to haematin. The oxidized haem initially binds to the specific haem-binding protein in plasma, haemopexin and the haem–haemopexin complexes are cleared by hepatocytes. After the haemopexin molecules are saturated, the haematin binds to albumin to form methaemalbumin which can be detected by Schumm's test. When haemoglobinaemia is present, some of the free Hb dissociates into dimers and the dimers pass through the glomerulus, thus causing haemoglobinuria. Some of the dimers are taken up by renal tubular cells and converted within the cells to haemosiderin. The haemosiderin may be detected in spun deposits of urine both inside shed tubular cells and extracellularly, using Perls' acid ferrocyanide reaction.

Morphological evidence of damage to red cells

A careful examination of a blood film may indicate the occurrence of haemolysis by revealing the presence of damaged or abnormal red cells such as microspherocytes, red cell fragments (schistocytes), sickled red cells or cells containing malarial parasites.

Reduced red cell lifespan

The most direct way to show that there is increased red cell destruction is to measure the red cell lifespan and demonstrate that it is shortened. The red cells are usually labelled with radioactive chromium (^{51}Cr) and reinjected into the patient. The survival of the labelled cells is then followed by taking blood samples at intervals and measuring their radioactivity (Fig. 3.1). By placing a γ-ray detector on the surface of the body over the spleen and liver, an indication of the main site of red cell destruction can also be obtained. When the ^{51}Cr accumulates predominantly in the spleen, splenectomy is usually followed by a partial or complete cure of the haemolytic process. Red cell lifespan measurements are rarely needed to diagnose haemolysis.

Laboratory evidence of increased erythropoietic activity

If evidence can be obtained of an increased rate of red cell production, this suggests that a haemolytic process is taking place, providing that there has been no loss of red cells through haemorrhage and the patient is not responding to therapy with iron, vitamin B$_{12}$ or folate. Two simple measurements can be used for assessing whether

Table 3.2 Evidence of increased erythropoietic activity.

Increased production
Peripheral blood
Reticulocytosis and erythroblastaemia; macrocytosis
Bone marrow
Erythroid hyperplasia; reduced myeloid/erythroid ratio
Bone
Changes in the skull and tubular bones

there is any increase in the rate of formation of red cells, namely, the reticulocyte count in the peripheral blood and the myeloid/erythroid ratio in the marrow (Table 3.2).

Reticulocytosis (increased reticulocyte count)

The number of reticulocytes in the blood is expressed either as a percentage of the total number of red cells or as an absolute number per litre of blood; in normal adults, the percentage is in the range of 0.5–3.0% and the absolute count is 20–100×10^9/L. In theory, the total number of reticulocytes in the circulation should be proportional to the rate of production of red cells, provided that there is no variation in the length of time that reticulocytes take to mature. In practice, reticulocytes released prematurely from the marrow following erythropoietin stimulation spend longer in the circulation than normal reticulocytes before they mature into adult cells. Nevertheless, an increase in the absolute reticulocyte count is an indication of increased erythropoietic activity and, in general, the higher the count, the greater the rate of delivery of viable red cells to the circulation. The reticulocyte percentage may increase up to 50% or more when erythropoietic activity is intense.

Erythroblastaemia and macrocytosis

Moderate or marked erythroid hyperplasia may be associated with the presence of occasional nucleated red cells (erythroblasts) in the circulation (erythroblastaemia). A high mean cell volume (MCV) that is unrelated to folate deficiency may also occur. This macrocytosis is related to the presence of a high proportion of reticulocytes in the blood; the reticulocytes formed during accelerated erythropoiesis are abnormally large and mature into rounded macrocytes. In addition, chronic erythroid hyperplasia imposes an increased demand for folate and if this is not met by adequate dietary intake, macrocytosis due to folate deficiency develops.

Erythroid hyperplasia and a reduced myeloid/erythroid ratio

A semiquantitative assessment of the degree of erythroid hyperplasia can be obtained by determining the myeloid/erythroid (M/E) ratio in the bone marrow. This is often defined as the ratio between the number of cells of the neutrophil series (including mature granulocytes) and the number of erythroblasts in bone marrow. The normal range for the M/E ratio in marrow smears from adults is two to eight (i.e. there are normally more cells of the neutrophil series than erythroblasts). A reduction of the M/E ratio is taken as evidence of erythroid hyperplasia, provided that the total number of cells of the neutrophil series can be assumed to be normal. Marrows showing erythroid hyperplasia are hypercellular, due to the replacement of fat cells by erythroblasts (Fig. 3.2). When erythroid hyperplasia is marked, fat cells may be virtually absent. Also, haemopoietic tissue may extend into marrow cavities that usually contain only fat, and extramedullary haemopoiesis may develop in the liver, spleen and lymph nodes.

Erythroid hyperplasia occurs not only in haemolytic states and after haemorrhage but also in megaloblastic and sideroblastic anaemias (where erythropoiesis is markedly ineffective, see p. 11), polycythaemia and erythroleukaemia.

Clinical features of haemolytic states

These result both from the increased red cell destruction and from the compensatory increase in erythropoietic activity. There may be pallor and mild jaundice. The prevalence of pigment stones in the gall bladder is increased; the stones may occasionally cause deep jaundice due to biliary obstruction. Splenomegaly is common. In patients

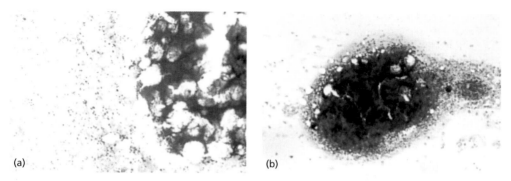

(a)

(b)

Figure 3.2 (a) A normocellular marrow fragment: about half its volume consists of haemopoietic cells (staining blue) and the remainder of unstained rounded fat cells. (b) A markedly hypercellular marrow fragment: virtually all the fat cells are replaced by haemopoietic cells.

with severe congenital haemolytic anaemias, the erythroid hyperplasia causes expansion of marrow cavities, thinning of cortical bone, bone deformities (e.g. frontal and parietal bossing) and, very occasionally, pathological fractures. These changes cause characteristic radiological abnormalities in the skull and other bones (Fig. 3.3). Occasionally, chronic leg ulcers develop over the malleoli.

Aplastic crises

Episodes of pure red cell aplasia, lasting about a week, may complicate the course of patients with chronic haemolytic anaemia. Erythroblasts virtually disappear from the marrow, the absolute reticulocyte count falls markedly (sometimes to zero) and the Hb falls rapidly. Such crises are often preceded by a febrile illness, with gastrointestinal symptoms, joint pains and, rarely, a maculopapular or erythematous rash, and are usually caused by infection of erythroid progenitor cells with parvovirus B19. Affected patients may have to be transfused with red cells urgently.

Diagnosis of haemolytic anaemia

There are two stages in the diagnosis of haemolytic anaemia:

1 The demonstration of a haemolytic state.
2 The determination of its aetiology.

The diagnosis of a haemolytic state is commonly made with reasonable confidence by the

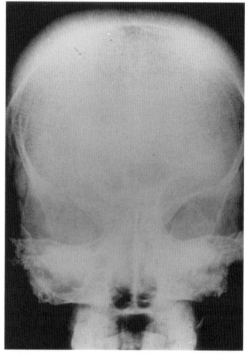

Figure 3.3 An X-ray of the skull of a patient with homozygous β-thalassaemia. The space between the abnormally thin tables of the skull bones is considerably widened due to erythroid hyperplasia. Bone trabeculae have developed at right angles to the tables giving a 'hair-on-end' appearance.

finding of an increase in both the reticulocyte count and the plasma bilirubin concentration, in a patient in whom alternative causes for these two abnormalities are excluded (e.g. haemorrhage and liver disease). Anaemia may or may not be present. Other findings indicating haemolysis have been discussed above (see Tables 3.1 and 3.2).

The next stage in diagnosis is to determine the nature of the disease causing the haemolysis. In approaching the diagnosis, it is useful to make a distinction between congenital abnormalities of the red cells on the one hand, and acquired abnormalities on the other. In the latter category, an agent acts on the red cell leading to its destruction (e.g. autoantibodies in autoimmune haemolytic anaemia). Congenital haemolytic anaemias may result from defects in one of three components of the red cell:

1 The cell membrane.
2 Enzyme systems concerned with the energy production that maintains the integrity of the cell.
3 Haemoglobin.

Congenital haemolytic anaemias

Defects of the red cell membrane

There is a submembranous filamentous protein meshwork that is attached to the inner surface of the red cell membrane, called the membrane cytoskeleton (Fig. 3.4). The four main proteins in this cytoskeleton are spectrin, actin, protein 4.1 and ankyrin. The cytoskeleton is important for maintaining the normal biconcave shape of the red cell.

Hereditary spherocytosis (HS)

The most common haemolytic anaemia due to a membrane defect is HS. About 60% of patients have mutations affecting the ankyrin gene leading to a decrease in ankyrin and secondary reductions in spectrin and protein 4.1. In other cases, there are various mutations in the genes for band 3, protein 4.2 or spectrin β- or α-chains. It has been proposed that these deficiencies lead to uncoupling of the cytoskeleton from the overlying lipid bilayer membrane and, consequently, to the release of bilayer lipids in the form of skeleton-free lipid vesicles. The loss of lipid results in a reduction of surface area and thus causes the older red cells to become microspherocytes. Repeated passage through the spleen aggravates the spherocytic change. Spherocytes are less deformable than normal red cells and are therefore retarded and eventually prevented from passing from the Billroth cords to the splenic sinusoids. The trapped cells are engulfed and destroyed by splenic macrophages, leading to a reduction in red cell survival.

The prevalence of the disease in North Europe is about one per 5000 of the population. The disease is usually inherited as an autosomal

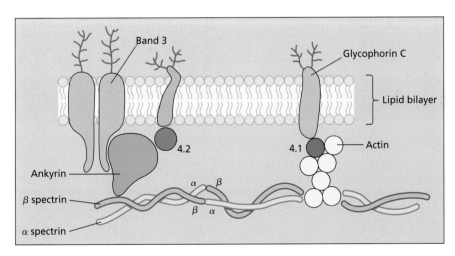

Figure 3.4 Schematic diagram of the red cell membrane cytoskeleton.

dominant character. Patients often give a family history of the condition, such as a parent or sibling who is known to have the disease or who has had recurrent anaemia, gall stones or a splenectomy.

The disease may present at any time from birth to old age and even *in utero*. There is a great difference in the severity of the disease: the Hb concentration varies from 4 to 5 g/dL to over 12 g/dL. In one study, half of the non-splenectomized patients were not anaemic.

Apart from anaemia, the main clinical findings in most patients are jaundice (more marked when there is coinheritance of Gilbert's disease in which hepatic conjugation of bilirubin is impaired) and an enlarged spleen. Most patients develop pigment stones in the gall bladder and 10–20% of those with intact spleens also develop acute cholecystitis or biliary obstruction.

Trivial viral illnesses may lead to episodes of increased red cell destruction during which the patient becomes more anaemic and jaundiced and frequently develops abdominal pain. Aplastic crises due to a temporary failure of red cell production by the bone marrow may also occur and are usually caused by parvovirus B19 (p. 28). Patients may present for the first time during a haemolytic or aplastic episode.

Megaloblastic anaemia due to folate deficiency is also occasionally found, as in other chronic haemolytic disorders. This results from an increased requirement for folate by the hyperactive bone marrow, and is especially found when the diet is inadequate.

Diagnosis

The cardinal clinical features are a family history, mild jaundice, pallor and splenomegaly. The laboratory findings of the greatest help in diagnosis are: the presence of spherocytes in the stained blood film (Fig. 3.5); an increased reticulocyte count; raised plasma bilirubin; increased osmotic fragility of the red cells; and a negative antiglobulin test (which excludes spherocytosis due to an autoantibody). The spherocytes appear as small densely staining cells and the percentage of spherocytes varies markedly from patient to patient. An important test which must always be carried out when spherocytes are infrequent is the osmotic fragility test. When normal red cells are suspended in a range of hypotonic saline solutions, they do not start to lyse until the saline concentration is reduced below 0.55 g/dL. In HS, the red cells are thicker than normal and some are already spherocytic, so that a smaller amount of fluid uptake than normal is sufficient to burst the cells (i.e. the cells have an increased osmotic fragility). Thus, these abnormal cells start to lyse when the saline concentration is as high as 0.6–0.8 g/dL.

Treatment

Severely anaemic children (Hb < 8 g/dL) should be subjected to splenectomy and moderately anaemic patients who are symptomatic or have complications such as gall stones should be considered for splenectomy. Since splenectomy, especially in children under the age of 5 years, is associated with an increased risk of fatal infections, particularly by encapsulated bacteria, it should be delayed until after the age of 5–10 years whenever possible. Furthermore, the risk of overwhelming infection should be minimized by the administration of pneumococcal and meningococcal vaccine and *Haemophilus influenzae* type b vaccine prior to splenectomy, and of prophylactic penicillin V post-splenectomy. Splenectomy

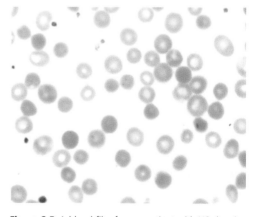

Figure 3.5 A blood film from a patient with HS showing several spherocytes.

regularly results in a rise in the Hb level to normal, the disappearance of jaundice and an increase of red cell lifespan to almost normal values. However, spherocytes persist.

Hereditary elliptocytosis and hereditary pyropoikilocytosis

Hereditary elliptocytosis, which affects one per 2500 of the population, is transmitted as an autosomal dominant trait. Characteristically, 25–90% of the red cells are oval, elliptical or rod-shaped (Fig. 3.6), whereas in a blood smear from a normal person only 0–5% of cells have this morphology. Most heterozygotes either do not have an appreciably shortened red cell lifespan or show evidence of a compensated haemolytic state. A few have a chronic symptomatic haemolytic anaemia. Homozygotes and compound heterozygotes usually have a severe haemolytic anaemia from infancy with microspherocytes and poikilocytes (hereditary pyropoikilocytosis).

Patients have various mutations affecting the spectrin genes or, less commonly, the protein 4.1 gene, which lead to abnormalities in the association of spectrin dimers into tetramers, partial or complete deficiency of protein 4.1, or a structurally abnormal protein 4.1. These mutations alter the elastic deformability of the membrane leading to a progressive failure to restore the circular shape of the red cell following repeated elliptical deformation in the microcirculation.

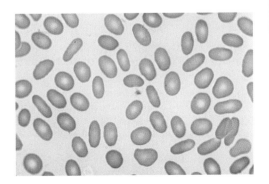

Figure 3.6 A blood film from a patient with hereditary elliptocytosis showing a high proportion of elliptical red cells.

Abnormalities of red cell enzymes

Haemolytic anaemias may also result from congenital abnormalities of the enzyme system concerned with energy transfer in glucose metabolism. The red cell requires a continuous supply of energy for the maintenance of membrane flexibility and cell shape, the regulation of sodium and potassium pumps, and the maintenance of Hb in the reduced ferrous form. The energy is obtained from glucose, which is converted to lactic acid mainly through the anaerobic glycolytic cycle (Embden–Meyerhof pathway). There is an alternative aerobic pathway, the pentose-phosphate shunt, starting with glucose-6-phosphate and requiring glucose-6-phosphate dehydrogenase (G6PD) as the initial enzyme (Fig. 3.7). Energy is transferred through the energy-rich compounds adenosine triphosphate (ATP), reduced nicotinamide-adenine dinucleotide

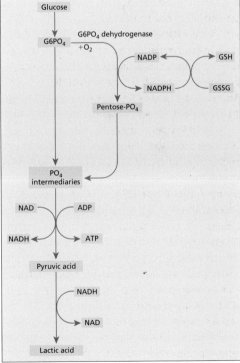

Figure 3.7 A schematic diagram of the pathway of glucose metabolism in the red cell, to show the important role of G6PD. A decreased activity of the enzyme leads to a deficiency of the reducing compounds NADPH and GSH.

(NADH), the related phosphorylated compound, NADPH and reduced glutathione (GSH).

The most common enzyme deficiency giving rise to a haemolytic anaemia is deficiency of G6PD, an enzyme within the pentose-phosphate shunt. Occasionally, deficiencies of other enzymes cause a congenital non-spherocytic haemolytic anaemia (e.g. deficiency of pyruvate kinase, an enzyme within the anaerobic glycolytic pathway).

G6PD deficiency

There are two types of normal G6PD enzyme. The most prevalent worldwide is designated type B. About 20% of healthy Africans have type A, which has normal enzyme activity and results from a single amino acid change from type B. It has been estimated that there may be as many as 400 million people in the world who have diminished red cell G6PD activity. The defective gene is present on the X-chromosome, and thus the clinical features of G6PD deficiency are mainly seen in males ($\bar{X}Y$, where $\bar{X}$ is the abnormal chromosome). Homozygous women ($\bar{X}\bar{X}$) are also clinically affected but such individuals are uncommon. The normal X-chromosome in a heterozygous woman ($\bar{X}X$) usually maintains sufficient G6PD activity to prevent clinical manifestations. The high prevalence of G6PD deficiency must have some Darwinian survival value and there is evidence indicating that deficiency gives some protection to the heterozygous female against *Plasmodium falciparum*; G6PD deficiency is common only in populations exposed for long periods to tertian malaria — heterozygous females with malaria have lower parasite counts in their red cells than normal women.

Deficiency of the enzyme is found in about 20% of blacks from west and central Africa and, to a varying extent, in southern Europe, the Middle East, India, Thailand and southern China. Deficiency is very rare in northern Europe. Virtually all of the 130 or so known variants of G6PD arise from single-point mutations within the coding region of the G6PD gene. Only two variants are common and these account for over 95% of cases. The most common is the African (or A–) type,

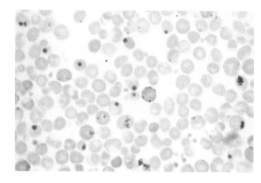

Figure 3.8 Rounded, darkly staining membrane-bound Heinz bodies consisting of denatured haemoglobin (supravital staining with methyl violet). The blood film shown is from a splenectomized patient with HbH disease and the Heinz bodies consist of denatured HbH. Similar inclusions of denatured HbA may be found in G6PD-deficient patients exposed to oxidant substances.

where G6PD function is reduced to about 10% of normal; in the less common Mediterranean type, the enzyme activity is reduced to 1–3%.

Low activities of G6PD result in low concentrations of the reducing compounds NADPH and GSH (see Fig. 3.7). The purpose of these compounds is to maintain Hb and other erythrocytic proteins in a reduced and active form. People with low levels of the enzymes are thus poorly protected against drugs that are oxidants. When oxidants enter the cell they first convert Hb to methaemoglobin and finally denature it so that it precipitates in the red cell in the form of rounded masses known as Heinz bodies (Fig. 3.8). These Heinz bodies (and the portion of the red cell membrane to which they become attached) are removed by splenic macrophages as the red cells pass through the spleen; the resulting inclusion-free cells stain densely, display unstained areas at their periphery ('bite' cells) (Fig. 3.9) and undergo extravascular haemolysis. Components of the red cell membrane may also undergo marked oxidation leading to intravascular haemolysis. Oxidant drugs that bring about this type of haemolytic anaemia include antimalarial drugs (e.g. primaquine, chloroquine, Fansidar, Maloprim), sulphonamides,

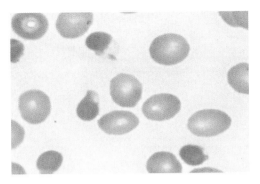

Figure 3.9 'Bite' cells in the blood film of a patient with G6PD deficiency who had received primaquine. These red cells are irregular in shape, are abnormally dense and show a poorly staining area just beneath part of the cell membrane (MGG stain).

nitrofurantoin, chloramphenicol, aspirin (high doses), phenacetin and vitamin K analogues.

A number of screening tests and assays for detecting G6PD deficiency are available. These are based on assessing the production of NADPH by red cells in the presence of an excess of glucose-6-phosphate. The NADPH is detected spectrophotometrically, or by its ability to reduce nitroblue tetrazolium (NBT) in the presence of an electron transfer agent, or by its ability to fluoresce in ultraviolet light.

A variety of clinical syndromes may be associated with G6PD variants that have reduced enzyme activity. These are outlined below.

Episodic acute haemolysis

Most of the time, patients with the two common G6PD variants (A– and Mediterranean types) are symptomless and have normal Hb concentrations with only a slight shortening of the red cell lifespan. Episodes of haemolytic anaemia develop during infections or following exposure to oxidant drugs and chemicals. Anaemia is maximal about 7–10 days after taking an oxidant. The extent of the fall in Hb concentration is partly dependent on the amount and nature of the drug being given, and partly on the extent of the reduction of enzyme activity. In patients with the Ã variant, after about 10 days and despite continuation of the drug, the Hb concentration rises again and may reach normal levels. This is because in these patients only the older cells have sufficiently low G6PD activities to be affected and destroyed by the drug. Heinz bodies may be demonstrated in circulating red cells during the early stages of haemolytic episodes. In patients with the Mediterranean type, in whom the average enzyme activity is very low, haemolysis may not be self-limiting.

Favism

Favism has been known for 2000 years or more. It is an acute haemolytic anaemia occurring after the ingestion of the broad bean (*Vicia fava*) in individuals with a deficiency of G6PD (commonly of the Mediterranean type). Favism usually affects children; severe anaemia develops rapidly and is often accompanied by haemoglobinuria. Fava beans contain two β-glycosides, vicine and convicine, which generate free radicals and consequently oxidize GSH and other red cell constituents.

> **Neonatal jaundice**
>
> Hyperbilirubinaemia, sometimes necessitating exchange transfusion, is occasionally found in G6PD-deficient neonates. The hyperbilirubinaemia may be due to hepatocyte dysfunction or oxidant damage to red cells. Affected individuals recover completely after the neonatal period but may develop episodic acute haemolysis (see above), during later life.
>
> **Congenital non-spherocytic haemolytic anaemia**
>
> Very rarely, the reduction in G6PD activity is so marked that there is substantial haemolysis and anaemia throughout life.

Abnormalities of the structure or synthesis of haemoglobin

Hb molecules present in fetal and postnatal life are composed of four polypeptide (globin) chains, two α-chains and two non-α-chains, which combine together to form a globular protein. Each globin chain is associated with a single haem group that can reversibly combine with O_2. Most of the Hb in a normal adult is called haemoglobin A (HbA) and contains two α- and two β-chains ($\alpha_2\beta_2$). Between 1.5% and 3.5% consists of haemoglobin A$_2$ ($\alpha_2\delta_2$) and less than 1% consists of haemoglobin F or fetal haemoglobin ($\alpha_2\gamma_2$).

Inherited abnormalities of Hb fall into two categories:

1 *Structural Hb variants (haemoglobinopathies)* in which there is an alteration in the amino acid sequence of a globin chain without a reduction in the rate of synthesis of the abnormal chain.
2 *Thalassaemia syndromes* in which there is a depression in the rate of synthesis of one of the globin chains.

> In the thalassaemia syndromes, the amino acid sequences of the globin chains are usually normal. However, a thalassaemic blood picture may sometimes arise from the presence of a structurally abnormal globin chain that is synthesized at a reduced rate (e.g. Hb Constant Spring and Hb Lepore) or of an abnormal Hb which is markedly unstable (e.g. Hb Indianapolis).

Structural haemoglobin variants

Over 700 abnormal Hbs shave been reported but most are rare and only a few lead to clinical or haematological manifestations. The majority of structural Hb variants are the consequence of a single-point mutation affecting one base triplet (codon) in a globin gene and therefore have a single amino acid substitution in the affected globin chain (e.g. HbS, HbE, HbC and HbD).

> If a single-point mutation affects the stop codon of the α-globin gene, the α-chains produced have extra amino acids at one end (e.g. in Hb Constant Spring). A few abnormal Hbs result from deletions of one or more base triplets or insertions of extra base triplets, consequently showing a loss of one or more amino acids or a gain of amino acids within a chain, respectively. An occasional variant results from fusion genes and contains hybrid chains made of parts of δ- and β-chains (in Hb Lepore) or γ- and β-chains (in Hb Kenya).

The spectrum of clinical and haematological abnormalities that may be caused by abnormal Hbs is summarized in Table 3.3. The most common structural Hb variant is haemoglobin S (HbS) and this is discussed in some detail below.

When the amino acid substitution results in an overall change in the charge of the molecule, its migration in a voltage gradient is altered and this can be demonstrated by standard electrophoretic techniques. The speed of migration is characteristic for each abnormal Hb (Fig. 3.10). Abnormal Hbs can also be detected by high-pressure liquid chromatography (HPLC).

Table 3.3 Different clinical and haematological abnormalities associated with some structural haemoglobin variants.

Variant	Clinical and haematological abnormalities
HbS	Recurrent painful crises (in adults) and chronic haemolytic anaemia; both related to sickling of red cells on deoxygenation*
HbC	Chronic haemolytic anaemia due to reduced red cell deformability on deoxygenation,* deoxygenated HbC is less soluble than deoxygenated HbA
Hb Köln, Hb Hammersmith	Spontaneous or drug-induced haemolytic anaemia due to instability of the Hb and consequent intracellular precipitation
HbM Boston, HbM Saskatoon	Cyanosis due to congenital methaemoglobinaemia as a consequence of a substitution near or in the haem pocket
Hb Chesapeake	Hereditary polycythaemia due to increased O$_2$ affinity
Hb Kansas	Anaemia and cyanosis due to decreased O$_2$ affinity
Hb Constant Spring, Hb Lepore, HbE	Thalassaemia-like syndrome due to decreased rate of synthesis of abnormal chain
Hb Indianapolis	Thalassaemia-like syndrome due to marked instability of Hb

Note: * Only in homozygotes.

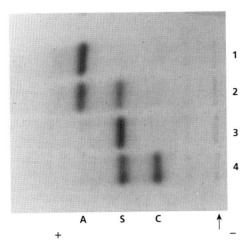

Figure 3.10 Electrophoresis of haemolysates on cellulose acetate (pH 8.5). The arrow marks the site of application of the haemolysate. (1) Normal adult. (2) Individual with sickle-cell trait; 35% of the Hb consists of HbS and most of the remainder is HbA. (3) Patient with sickle-cell anaemia; most of the Hb is S and there is no A. (4) Double heterozygote for HbS and HbC. This results in a disease which is usually milder than that in homozygotes for HbS.

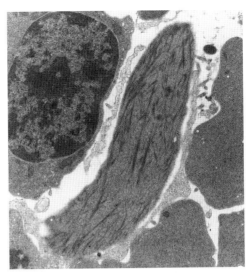

Figure 3.11 Electron micrograph of a sickled red cell from a homozygote for HbS showing fibres of polymerized deoxygenated HbS running along the long axis of the cell.

Haemoglobin S

In this Hb, the charged glutamic acid residue in position 6 of the normal β-chain is replaced by an uncharged valine molecule. This results in deoxygenated HbS being 50 times less soluble than deoxygenated HbA. The deoxygenated HbS molecules initially polymerize without forming fibres and subsequently polymerize into long fibres (tactoids) (Fig. 3.11) which deform the red cell into the typical sickle shape (Fig. 3.12). Red cells from heterozygotes for HbS sickle at much lower P_{O_2} values than those from homozygotes, and do not usually sickle *in vivo*.

The gene for HbS occurs particularly in a wide area across tropical Africa, in some countries bordering on the northern shores of the Mediterranean, and in parts of the Middle East and southern India (Fig. 3.13). The prevalence of this gene in these areas varies from very low values up to 40% of the population. In black Americans, the prevalence is 8%. The distribution of the HbS gene corresponds to areas in which falciparum malaria has been endemic; the persistence of this

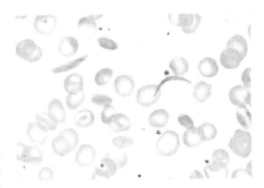

Figure 3.12 Two sickle-shaped red cells with pointed ends and some partially sickled red cells from the blood film of a patient with sickle-cell anaemia (homozygote for HbS).

potentially lethal gene in high frequency in these areas results from the fact that heterozygotes die less frequently from severe falciparum malaria during early childhood than children with only HbA.

Sickle-cell trait

Heterozygotes (one gene for HbA and one for HbS) are described as having sickle-cell trait. Their red cells contain between 20% and 45% HbS, the rest being mainly HbA. Heterozygotes do not have 50% HbS mainly because mutant

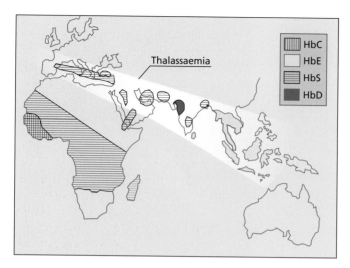

Thalassaemia

HbC
HbE
HbS
HbD

Figure 3.13 Distribution of the genes for the major Hb variants (S, E, C, D) and thalassaemia.

β-chains (β^S) have a lower affinity than normal β-chains to associate with α-chains. Individuals with sickle-cell trait are haematologically normal and are usually asymptomatic. However, spontaneous haematuria may occur occasionally and renal papillary necrosis rarely. Furthermore, there is often an impaired ability to concentrate urine in older individuals. The red cells do not sickle in the trait until the O_2 saturation falls below 40%, a level that is rarely reached in venous blood. Painful crises (see p. 37) and splenic infarction have occurred in severely hypoxic individuals.

Sickle-cell anaemia

Homozygotes for HbS are described as having sickle-cell anaemia. Their red cells contain 80% or more HbS and no HbA; the remainder is mainly fetal Hb. The cells sickle at the O_2 tension normally found in venous blood. Initially, there are cycles of sickling and reversal of sickling as the red cells are repeatedly deoxygenated and oxygenated within the circulation. Eventually, irreversibly sickled cells are formed. Both unsickled and sickled red cells containing deoxygenated HbS are less deformable than normal red cells and suffer mainly extravascular haemolysis. The increased rigidity of the cells may cause them to become jammed in and obstruct small and, occasionally, medium-sized blood vessels, thus causing tissue infarction. The adhesion of sickled cells to activated neutrophils and endothelial cells plays an

Table 3.4 Clinical manifestations of sickle-cell anaemia.

Chronic haemolytic anaemia and consequent cholelithiasis

Splenic sequestration syndrome; rarely, hepatic sequestration

Acute chest syndrome

Cerebral infarction, TIA, intracranial haemorrhage

Widespread painful vasoocclusive crises

Bone infarction (osteonecrosis)

Osteomyelitis (*Salmonella, Staphylococcus*)

Chronic leg ulcers

Priapism

Chronic pulmonary disease and pulmonary hypertension

Hyposthenuria, haematuria, proteinuria, chronic renal failure

Pregnancy: increased peripartum fetal loss, preterm births, babies small for gestational age

Aplastic crises due to parvovirus infection

Proliferative sickle retinopathy (more common in HbSC disease)

important role in vaso-occlusion. Symptoms due to infarction are not present continuously but occur in episodes.

There is a chronic haemolytic anaemia (Table 3.4), with the Hb usually varying between 6 and 9 g/dL; the symptoms of anaemia are milder than expected from the Hb levels as HbS has a reduced affinity for O_2 (the O_2 dissociation curve is shifted to the right) (p. 2). The haemolysis may lead to the formation of pigment gall stones. Different tissues are liable to infarction at different ages so that the clinical picture varies markedly with age. Furthermore, some patients are only mildly affected, having few or no infarctive episodes at any age. In some of these patients, the mildness of the disease is related to the coinheritance of one or two α-thalassaemia genes (which reduces the mean cell Hb concentration (MCHC)) or a gene for the hereditary persistence of HbF.

A characteristic feature of sickle-cell anaemia in infancy and early childhood is dactylitis, or the hand–foot syndrome, resulting from occlusion of the nutrient arteries to the metacarpals and metatarsals (Fig. 3.14). There is a painful, non-erythematous and often symmetrical swelling of the hands and feet, lasting 10–14 days. Infants and young children may also develop a life-threatening acute splenic sequestration syndrome. Here there is rapid and extensive trapping of red cells in the spleen leading to profound anaemia, massive splenomegaly, reduced blood volume and hypovolaemic shock. Other cases may develop hepatic sequestration. Sickle-cell anaemia patients show an increased susceptibility to fulminant bacterial infections, especially in the first 3 years of life, apparently due to a combination of hyposplenism (despite the splenomegaly) and an abnormality in opsonization.

The acute chest syndrome (acute febrile illness with dyspnoea, chest pain and radiological changes) is the most common cause of death after the age of 2 years; this syndrome results from a combination of pulmonary infection, infarction and sequestration. Strokes due to cerebral infarction also occur in 10–15% of cases, especially between the ages of 3 and 10. Transcranial Doppler studies at the ages of 2 and 3 allows identification of children at high risk.

In older children and adults, recurrent episodes of widespread microvascular occlusion lead to painful crises. These usually consist of attacks of pain affecting the bones and large joints of all four limbs and the back. The crises are accompanied by low-grade fever and may last from a few days to a few weeks. Occasionally the pain may be felt predominantly in one limb or in the chest or abdomen. Patients in this age group also suffer from larger infarcts affecting the bones (leading to avascular necrosis of the heads of the femora or humeri and of the diaphyses of long bones). The spleen is usually palpable in children, but it atrophies from repeated infarction and is usually not felt in adults.

Other clinical features include *Salmonella* infection of necrotic bone (osteomyelitis), chronic leg ulcers (Fig. 3.15) and priapism. Some patients develop chronic pulmonary disease or pulmonary hypertension. Patients are unable to concentrate urine normally from an early age and other tubular defects may be found. Occasionally, painless haematuria develops due to small medullary infarcts or papillary necrosis. Glomerular

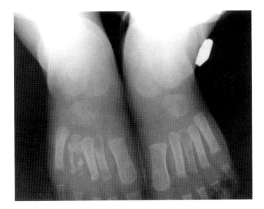

Figure 3.14 An X-ray of the feet of a child with sickle-cell anaemia 2 weeks after the onset of hand–foot syndrome, showing necrosis of the right fourth metatarsal.

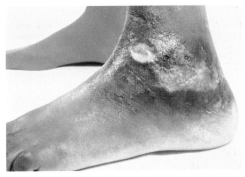

Figure 3.15 A chronic leg ulcer with increased pigmentation of the surrounding skin in a woman with sickle-cell anaemia.

dysfunction may lead to proteinuria. Rarely, the nephrotic syndrome may develop in adults and progress to renal failure. Chronic renal failure is encountered especially after the age of 40 years and is caused by a combination of cortical and medullary infarction, glomerular sclerosis, tubular damage and infection. Pregnancy may be associated with a worsening of symptoms and there is an increased occurrence of peripartum fetal loss and premature or low birth weight babies.

A proliferative sickle retinopathy (PSR) may develop and could lead to blindness from vitreous haemorrhage and retinal detachment; PSR is more common in double heterozygotes for HbS and HbC (i.e. in HbSC disease) than in sickle-cell anaemia. Aplastic crises due to parvovirus infection may occur (p. 28) as may an aggravation of the anaemia due to a secondary folate deficiency (p. 27).

Diagnosis

Many patients with sickle-cell anaemia have at least a few sickled cells in their blood film (see Fig. 3.12). The diagnosis is made by finding: (i) a positive result with a screening test for HbS; (ii) a single major band moving in the position of HbS on electrophoresis both at an alkaline and acid pH (see Fig. 3.10); and (iii) the sickle-cell trait in both parents. The screening tests for HbS-containing red cells are based on the decreased solubility of deoxygenated HbS; they involve the development of turbidity after addition to a lysis buffer containing a reducing agent such as sodium dithionite (sickle solubility test). Heterozygotes for HbS also give a positive result with these screening tests but do not have sickled cells on their blood films, and show a mixture of HbA and HbS on electrophoresis.

Treatment

Principles of management of sickle-cell anaemia include:

1 Immunization with pneumococcal, *Haemophilus influenzae* type b (Hib) and meningococcal vaccine and treatment with prophylactic penicillin V to minimize the risk from fulminant infections. Non-immune patients should also receive hepatitis B vaccine in case multiple transfusions are required.

2 Administration of folic acid daily to prevent secondary folate deficiency.

3 Avoidance of factors precipitating painful crises such as dehydration, hypoxia, circulatory stasis and cooling of the skin.

4 Active treatment for bacterial infections that may precipitate or have precipitated crises.

5 Treatment of painful crises with oral or intravenous fluids and analgesics, including opiates when necessary (e.g. continuous subcutaneous infusion of diamorphine).

6 Early detection of the acute chest syndrome (blood gas measurements and chest X-ray) and the administration of O_2 by mask in hypoxic patients.

7 Blood transfusion in certain circumstances. Transfusion is indicated for visceral sequestration and aplastic crises. Exchange transfusions are useful in certain situations, particularly in severe acute chest syndrome, in priapism, when there is evidence of neurological damage, when transcranial Doppler studies indicate that the risk of stroke is high and when crises occur very frequently. In the latter situation, exchange transfusion should be followed by regular blood transfusion to keep the HbS level below 40%; patients who are regularly transfused for prolonged periods (>1–2 years) must receive desferrioxamine (DFO) to prevent iron overload. Regular transfusion may be required during pregnancy in patients with frequent crises or a poor obstetric history.

8 In patients having frequent severe crises (three or more per year), prolonged therapy with hydroxyurea increases HbF production and causes a significant reduction in the incidence of such crises. Increased γ-chain synthesis has a beneficial effect because it leads to the formation of $\alpha_2\gamma\beta^S$ molecules which do not participate in polymer formation with $\alpha_2\beta^S_2$ on deoxygenation.

A number of severely affected children with sickle-cell anaemia have been treated by bone marrow transplantation from an HLA-identical sibling donor. The transplantation-related mortality is 5–10% and the disease-free survival is 80–90%.

Prognosis

There is a high infant mortality rate, especially when the quality of health care or compliance with advice is poor. With the use of prophylactic penicillin V (from 2 months up to at least 5 years) deaths due to pneumococcal sepsis (meningitis, pneumonia, septicaemia) have been reduced. Awareness and prompt treatment of the acute splenic sequestration syndrome has lead to a reduction of early deaths due to this cause. The acute chest syndrome is a common cause of death both in children and adults, with mortality rates between 5% and 10%. Adults may die of organ failure. The median survival is reduced, being about 50 years.

Haemoglobins E and C

Both HbE and HbC result from single amino acid substitutions in the β-chains.

HbE is very common in south-east Asia and is found in about 50% of the population in some parts of Thailand. Heterozygotes have about 20–30% HbE, are asymptomatic, and are usually not anaemic. They have a low MCV because the single base substitution in the β-globin gene creates an alternative splicing site in the primary mRNA transcript and, consequently, there is reduced production of mature mRNA for β^E-chains and reduced β^E-chain synthesis. Their blood films may contain a few target cells. Homozygotes are characterized by mild anaemia, a low MCV and many circulating target cells.

HbC is confined to people of west African extraction, being present in 7% and 22% of the population in Nigeria and northern Ghana, respectively. Heterozygotes have 30–40% HbC, are asymptomatic and non-anaemic, having 6–40% target cells in their blood. Homozygotes have a mild anaemia, low MCV, splenomegaly and many target cells (Fig. 3.16).

Thalassaemia

The thalassaemias are broadly divided into two main groups, the α-thalassaemias and the

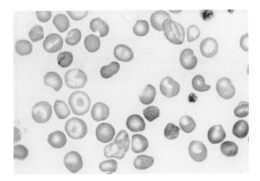

Figure 3.16 Target cells in the blood film of a homozygote for HbC.

β-thalassaemias, depending on whether the defect lies in the synthesis of α- or β-globin chains, respectively.

α-Thalassaemias

The α-thalassaemias are seen with greatest frequency in south-east Asia (Thailand, the Malay Peninsula and Indonesia) and west Africa, the prevalence in these countries being 20–30%. They are also seen in southern Europe and the Middle East and sporadic cases have been reported in most racial groups. There are two closely linked α-globin genes on chromosome 16 and thus four α-globin genes per cell. In most patients with α-thalassaemia syndromes, the primary biochemical defect is a deletion of one, two, three or all four of the α-globin genes. However, dysfunctional rather than completely deleted genes are also occasionally found; these are caused by partial deletions or non-deletional defects (usually a single base change). The manifestations of α-thalassaemia depend on the number of genes deleted in a particular individual. Deletion of one or two genes causes an asymptomatic condition with minor haematological changes; deletion of three and four genes causes HbH disease and Hb Bart's hydrops fetalis syndrome, respectively. There are two main varieties of abnormal chromosome (Fig. 3. 17). In the first, one of the two genes on a chromosome is deleted (α^+-thalassaemia determinant); in the second, both genes are deleted

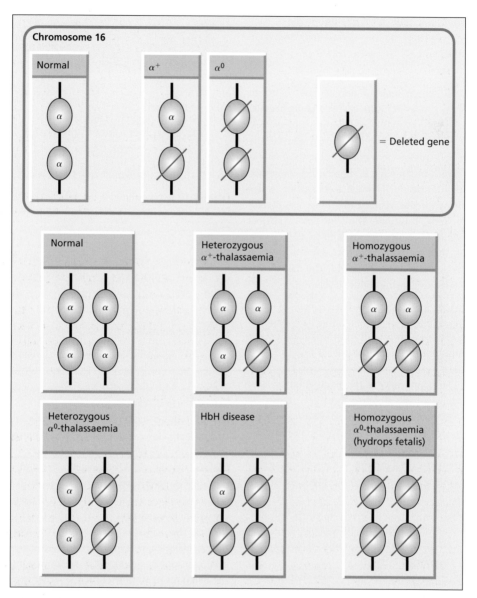

Figure 3.17 A diagram to show how the two forms of abnormal chromosome 16 (α^+ and α^0) are arranged to give the different forms of α-thalassaemia. Homozygotes for α^0-thalassaemia suffer from Hb Bart's hydrops fetalis syndrome.

(α^0-thalassaemia determinant). Both the α^0-thalassaemia and the α^+-thalassaemia determinants are found in south-east Asia and the Mediterranean region. The main type of α-thalassaemia determinant found in west Africa, the Middle East, India and the Pacific Islands is α^+; α^0 is very rare. In populations in which the

α^0-thalassaemia determinant is rare, HbH disease is rare and Hb Bart's hydrops fetalis syndrome is not found. In northern Thailand, where both the α^+ and α^0 determinants are particularly common, 0.4% of deliveries are stillbirths due to Hb Bart's hydrops fetalis syndrome and HbH disease is found in about 1% of the population.

α^+-Thalassaemia trait (deletion of one α-globin gene)

This condition is seen when the α^+-thalassaemia determinant is present on only one of the number 16 chromosomes (i.e. in heterozygotes for the α^+ determinant). Patients are asymptomatic but may be slightly anaemic. About 15% show slight reductions in MCV and mean cell Hb (MCH).

α^0-Thalassaemia trait (deletion of both α-globin genes on one chromosome 16)

This is seen in heterozygotes for the α^0-thalassaemia determinant. The Hb is either normal or slightly reduced and the MCV and MCH are usually reduced. (Similar haematological changes are seen in homozygotes for the α^+-thalassaemia determinant who also have two deleted α-globin genes.)

Haemoglobin H disease (deletion of three genes)

This chronic haemolytic anaemia results from the presence of both the α^+- and α^0-thalassaemia determinants. α-chains are produced at very low rates and there is a considerable excess of β-chains, which combine to form tetramers (β_4). This tetramer is known as HbH. HbH is unstable and precipitates as the erythrocytes get older, forming rigid Heinz bodies (see Fig. 3.8) that are removed during the passage of affected red cells through the spleen. The damage to the membrane brought about by this removal results in a shortened red cell lifespan. The clinical picture of HbH disease is very variable. Most patients are moderately affected with a condition similar to β-thalassaemia intermedia, some are more severely affected and others are only mildly affected and live almost normal lives. Splenomegaly is seen in most patients. The Hb concentration is usually between 7 and 11 g/dL but may be as low as 3–4 g/dL; the red cells are hypochromic and show variation in size and shape (Fig. 3.18). Both the MCV and MCH are reduced.

Hb Bart's hydrops fetalis syndrome (deletion of four genes)

This occurs when there is homozygosity for the α^0-thalassaemia determinant. No α-chains can be

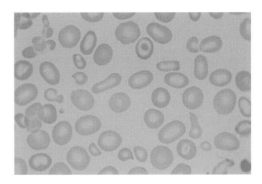

Figure 3.18 Blood film from a patient with HbH disease showing microcytosis, hypochromia, anisocytosis and poikilocytosis.

formed and the predominant chain synthesized is the γ-chain, which forms tetramers (γ_4, Hb Bart's). There is persistence in the fetus of the embryonic Hb, Hb Portland ($\zeta_2\gamma_2$). Intrauterine death followed by a stillbirth usually occurs between 25 and 40 weeks of gestation, or the baby dies very shortly after birth.

β-Thalassaemias

The prevalence of β-thalassaemia trait in southern Europe, south-east Asia and Africa is about 10–30%, 5% and 1.5%, respectively. The trait is also frequently seen in the Middle East, India, Pakistan and southern China. It has been suggested that the high prevalence of the β-thalassaemia gene in these regions results from the gene bestowing a protective effect against *Plasmodium falciparum* on heterozygotes.

The β-thalassaemias result from more than 200 different genetic abnormalities affecting the β-gene or the upstream promoter regions flanking the β-gene or the β-locus control region (p. 2); the prevalence of particular abnormalities varies between different races. When the β-chain genes are affected, they are usually not completely deleted but often show single nucleotide substitutions or additions, or small deletions. Patients in whom the genetic abnormality causes an absence of β-chain production are described as having β^0-thalassaemia, and those in whom the abnormality causes a reduction in the rate of

β-chain production are described as having β^+-thalassaemia. The β^0 type predominates in India and Pakistan, the β^+ type predominates in Sardinia and Cyprus; both types are found in Greece, the Middle East and Thailand.

Mutations in the coding region of the β-gene may disrupt the normal reading frame (frame-shifts) or introduce a premature termination codon (non-sense mutations). Mutations may also affect the initiator codon, regions involved in RNA processing, the polyadenylation site or the CAP site (p. 3). In some β-thalassaemia mutations, no mRNA is produced at all, in others there is a reduced production, and in some, structurally and/or functionally abnormal mRNA is transcribed and sometimes translated into structurally abnormal (truncated) β-chains that do not form viable tetramers.

Heterozygous β-thalassaemia

Most affected subjects are asymptomatic. The Hb concentration is either normal (thalassaemia minima) or slightly reduced (thalassaemia minor), the red cell count is high and the MCV is usually low. The Romanowsky-stained blood film shows microcytosis, target cells and red cells with basophilic stippling (i.e. several fine or coarse bluish-black granules consisting of aggregated ribosomes). The HbA$_2$ level is raised to 3.5–7.0% and half the cases show slightly increased HbF levels, which are in the range 1–5%. Serum iron, serum transferrin and serum ferritin are normal in the absence of coexisting iron deficiency.

Homozygous β-thalassaemia

This condition causes one of two syndromes, one characterized by severe anaemia usually developing between the 2nd and 12th months of life (β-thalassaemia major), and the other by moderate anaemia presenting after the age of 1–2 years (β-thalassaemia intermedia).

The inability to produce β-chains leads to the presence of an excess of α-chains (globin chain imbalance) in early and late polychromatic erythroblasts. Some of the excess α-chains precipitate within the cells and both the free and precipitated α-chains impair various cellular functions. Many of the precipitate-containing erythroblasts are eventually phagocytosed and degraded by bone marrow macrophages (ineffective erythropoiesis). There is also a considerably shortened survival of free α-globin and precipitate-containing red cells that enter the circulation so that the anaemia results from a combination of inadequate Hb synthesis, ineffective erythropoiesis and peripheral haemolysis. The response to the anaemia and ineffective erythropoiesis is an enormous erythroid hyperplasia that results in skeletal changes mainly affecting the skull, long bones and hands.

β-thalassaemia major (Cooley's anaemia)

This disease does not present at birth since production of fetal Hb, $\alpha_2\gamma_2$, is not affected. The infant becomes profoundly anaemic (Hb concentration 2.5–6.5 g/dL) and mildly jaundiced after the first few months of life, at the time when HbA should be replacing HbF. There is also failure to thrive, abdominal enlargement due to hepatosplenomegaly, and recurrent fever. If a transfusion programme is not instituted, growth is retarded, the abdomen becomes more enlarged, muscle development is poor and various skeletal deformities due to the gross expansion of erythropoietic tissue appear. The skeletal changes cause the typical 'thalassaemic' facies with frontal and parietal bossing, enlargement of the maxillary bones causing severe dental deformities and malocclusion of the teeth, and depression of the bridge of the nose. The long bones and bones of the hands show thinning of the cortex. Fractures of the long bones may occur. An X-ray of the skull shows enlargement of the diploic spaces and radiating striations in the subperiosteal bone ('hair-on-end' appearance) (see Fig. 3.3).

The excessive red cell destruction causes considerable enlargement of the spleen, and this itself may aggravate the anaemia due to increased pooling of red cells in that organ, an expanded plasma volume and secondary hypersplenism with a further shortening of red cell lifespan. The hypersplenism also causes neutropenia and thrombocytopenia.

Iron absorption from the gut is increased, and this, together with the regular blood transfusions (each unit of blood contains 200 mg iron) causes iron overload which, in the absence of long-term iron chelation therapy, usually leads to death between the ages of 10 and 20 years. Iron deposition causes cirrhosis of the liver, diabetes mellitus and myocardial damage leading to fatal arrhythmias or congestive cardiac failure. The iron deposition also causes endocrine dysfunction; this leads to a failure to grow normally during puberty and a delay or failure in the development of secondary sexual characteristics. With regular iron chelation therapy 90% of cases live into their late 30s or early 40s.

Diagnosis of β-thalassaemia major

The peripheral blood contains microcytic hypochromic red cells, which also vary greatly in size and shape and target cells (Fig. 3.19). Electrophoresis of Hb shows only or mainly HbF. There is an absence or reduction of HbA, depending on whether the abnormal genes are of the β^0 or β^+ type. The serum iron concentration is high, the serum transferrin concentration is usually slightly low and the transferrin saturation is high. The serum ferritin level is increased, roughly in proportion to the extent of iron overload.

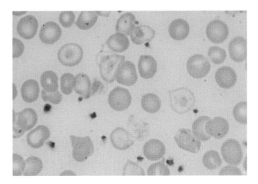

Figure 3.19 Peripheral blood film of a regularly transfused patient with homozygous β-thalassaemia showing poorly haemoglobinized target cells and hypochromic red cells together with many transfused normochromic normocytic red cells.

Treatment of β-thalassaemia major

Therapy centres on regular transfusions, about every 3–5 weeks, so that the pre-transfusion Hb concentration is always maintained at 9–10 g/dL or above with a post-transfusion Hb concentration of 13–14 g/dL. With this treatment, children grow and mature normally and lead normal lives. If the spleen is considerably enlarged and there is clear evidence that it is also trapping the transfused red cells and increasing transfusion requirements, splenectomy is carried out. An important aspect of treatment is the reduction of tissue damage due to secondary iron overload by the daily administration of the iron-chelating agent, DFO. This agent is given subcutaneously overnight using a portable pump and has been shown to limit iron accumulation and prolong life. However, it is costly and lack of compliance is common. Serious side effects are not frequent and include *Yersinia enterocolitica* infections, lens opacity, retinopathy and high-tone deafness. An oral iron chelator deferiprone (L1) is now available; it is less effective and much more toxic than DFO but compliance is better. The use of L1 in combination with DFO results in a synergistic increase in iron excretion as well as a reduction in L1-related toxicity. A major advantage of L1 is that its regular use reduces cardiac iron overload. A new oral chelator (Exjade) with limited side effects is now available.

Many patients have been treated with bone marrow transplants from an HLA-matched sibling or parent. The transplant-related mortality is high in older patients compared with children under the age of 17 and when the extent of iron overload and consequent tissue damage is substantial. The thalassaemia-free survival in children who have had regular iron chelation therapy and who do not have hepatic portal fibrosis is around 85%. This figure for adults especially with substantial iron overload or chronic active hepatitis is around 60%.

Genetic counselling and antenatal diagnosis of β-thalassaemia major

When a pregnant woman is found to have an abnormality in the synthesis or structure of Hb, her partner must also be investigated. If there is a risk of a serious clinical disease in the offspring, antenatal diagnosis should be offered. Antenatal diagnosis can be made early during pregnancy from an analysis of chorionic villous DNA (at 9–12 weeks) or amniocyte DNA (at 13–16 weeks) or later using DNA from blood obtained from an 18- to 20-week-old fetus. Several methods have been employed over the years. The two methods most widely used today are based on amplifying DNA 1 million times or more using the polymerase chain reaction (PCR). The first uses allele-specific primers that only amplify particular alleles (the amplification refractory mutation system, ARMS). The second uses consensus primers that amplify all the alleles and a particular allele is detected using allele-specific oligonucleotide probes. An early method was to analyze reticulocytes from fetal blood for β-chain production; the diagnosis of homozygous β-thalassaemia was made when β-chain production was absent or markedly reduced.

β-thalassaemia intermedia

Most patients with this condition are reasonably well and require transfusions only during intercurrent infections. Clinical features include skeletal deformities (see p. 42), splenomegaly (which may become sufficiently marked to require splenectomy), formation of masses of extramedullary haemopoietic tissue (which may cause pressure symptoms), recurrent leg ulcers and haemosiderosis in adult life due to increased iron absorption. The clinical picture of β-thalassaemia intermedia is less severe than that of β-thalassaemia major because the extent of globin chain imbalance (see p. 42) is smaller in the former than in the latter. The reduced chain imbalance may be a consequence of homozygosity for a 'mild' β-thalassaemia gene, homozygosity for Hb Lepore or $\delta\beta$-thalassaemia, heterozygosity for both β-thalassaemia and $\delta\beta$-thalassaemia, or heterozygosity for both β-thalassaemia and HbE. Alternatively, the extent of chain imbalance in homozygous β-thalassaemia may be reduced by coinheritance of one or two α-thalassaemia genes or by increased γ-chain synthesis (e.g. caused by a mutation leading to hereditary persistence of HbF). As has been mentioned, the clinical picture of thalassaemia intermedia is also found in HbH disease (an α-thalassaemia syndrome).

Acquired haemolytic anaemias

Red cells may be destroyed either by immunological or by non-immunological mechanisms.

Immune haemolytic anaemias

In these conditions, red cells react with antibody with or without complement activation and are consequently destroyed. IgG-coated red cells interact with the Fc receptors on macrophages and are then either completely or partially phagocytosed. When the phagocytosis is partial, the unphagocytosed part of the cell may detach from the macrophage and circulate as a spherocyte. Red cells that are also coated with the activated complement component C3 interact with C3 receptors on macrophages and are usually completely phagocytosed. In most instances where complement is activated, the cascade sequence only proceeds as far as C3 deposition on the cell surface. In a few instances, activation of complement is more intense and proceeds as far as deposition of the membrane attack complex (C5–C9), which results in intravascular haemolysis.

The immune haemolytic anaemias may be due to alloantibodies (antibodies produced by an individual that reacts with antigens of another individual of the same species) as in haemolytic transfusion reactions (p. 172) and haemolytic disease of the newborn (p. 177) or autoantibodies (antibodies formed against one or more antigenic constituents of the individuals own tissues) as in autoimmune haemolytic anaemias (AIHAs) and some drug-related haemolytic anaemias. In paroxysmal nocturnal haemoglobinuria (PNH), there is an acquired defect in the red cell membrane which leads to complement-mediated haemolysis.

Autoimmune haemolytic anaemias

A classification of the AIHAs is given in Table 3.5. The antibody found may be of two types: 'warm' antibody or 'cold' antibody. A 'warm' antibody reacts best with the red cell at 37°C and does not bring about agglutination. A 'cold' antibody reacts best only at temperatures below 32°C (usually

Table 3.5 Classification of AIHAs.

Caused by warm-reactive antibodies
Idiopathic
Secondary (chronic lymphocytic leukaemia, lymphoma,
   systemic lupus erythematosus (SLE), some drugs)
Caused by cold-reactive antibodies
Cold haemagglutinin disease
Idiopathic
Secondary (*Mycoplasma pneumoniae* infection,
   infectious mononucleosis, lymphomas)
Paroxysmal cold haemoglobinuria
Idiopathic
Secondary (some viral infections, congenital and
   tertiary syphilis)

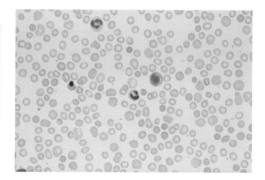

Figure 3.20 Blood film from a patient with idiopathic AIHA (warm-reactive antibody). In addition to several microspherocytes, the photomicrograph shows one erythroblast.

below 15°C) and usually agglutinates the red cells. The clinical picture associated with the two types is different.

AIHA with warm-reactive antibodies

Patients are usually over the age of 50 years. In the idiopathic condition haemolysis dominates the clinical picture, and no evidence can be found of any other disease. In the secondary condition, the haemolysis is associated with a primary disease such as chronic lymphocytic leukaemia or systemic lupus erythematosus (SLE). Fifty to seventy percent of 'warm' autoantibodies show specificity for the Rh antigen system and some of the remainder for other blood group antigen systems.

Symptoms are unrelated to ambient temperature. The clinical presentation is extremely variable. Some patients are very ill with an acute onset of severe anaemia; others have few or no symptoms and a mild chronic anaemia or even a compensated haemolytic state. Mild jaundice is common and splenomegaly is almost always found.

Haematological findings include anaemia, spherocytosis (Fig. 3.20), reticulocytosis, erythroblastaemia and neutrophil leucocytosis. IgG, complement components, or both can usually be detected on the red cells using a direct antiglobulin test.

In most patients, the haemolysis can be reduced by treatment with prednisolone, which is initially given in high doses. If there is no response to steroids, or if the reduction in haemolysis is not maintained when the dose of steroids is decreased, splenectomy or immunosuppressive therapy with drugs such as vinca alkaloids, azathioprine or cyclophosphamide should be tried and may be beneficial. High-dose intravenous immunoglobulin has also been used but is consistently less effective than in idiopathic autoimmune thrombocytopenic purpura (ITP). In patients with severe anaemia, the least incompatible ABO- and Rh-matched blood should be transfused.

Cold haemagglutinin disease

Since cold antibody only reacts with red cells at a temperature below about 32°C, symptoms are worse during cold weather; skin temperature frequently falls well below 32°C when exposed to the cold. Exposure to cold provokes acrocyanosis (coldness, purplish discoloration and numbness of fingers, toes, ear lobes and the nose). This symptom is due to the formation of agglutinates of red cells in the vessels of the skin. Cold antibody attached to red cells also activates the complement system and leads to red cell lysis and, consequently, to haemoglobinaemia and haemoglobinuria.

Blood films made at room temperature show large red cell agglutinates (Fig. 3.21). The cold agglutinin in chronic idiopathic CHAD (cold haemagglutinin disease) is usually a monoclonal

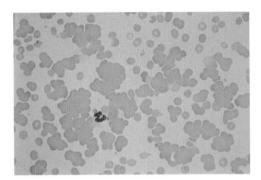

Figure 3.21 Numerous red cell agglutinates on a blood film from a patient with idiopathic CHAD.

IgM antibody, normally with anti-I specificity. The anti-I titre at 4°C may be as high as 1:2000 to 1:500,000 (normal, 1:10–40). (I and i are carbohydrate antigens expressed on red cells; adult red cells contain more I than i determinants.)

Rarely, patients with Mycoplasma pneumonia or infectious mononucleosis may develop acute self-limiting CHAD due to the production of polyclonal IgM antibodies with anti-I or anti-i specificity, respectively.

Paroxysmal cold haemoglobinuria

This rare disease is caused by an IgG antibody with anti-P specificity (P is a glycolipid red cell antigen). This antibody is capable of binding complement and is called the Donath–Landsteiner antibody. Patients suffer from acute episodes of marked haemoglobinuria due to severe intravascular haemolysis when exposed to the cold. The diagnosis is based on serological studies demonstrating the presence of this particular antibody. A rapid screening test consists of incubating the patient's red cells and serum at 4°C and then warming the mixture to 37°C. Antibody and early complement components bind to red cells at 4°C but lysis occurs only on warming to 37°C (Donath–Landsteiner test). An acute transient form associated with a viral infection affects children. The chronic form is usually seen in adults with syphilis.

Paroxysmal nocturnal haemoglobinuria (PNH)

This is an acquired disease in which an abnormal clone of haemopoietic cells derived from an abnormal haemopoietic stem cell gives rise to erythrocytes, leucocytes and platelets with defects in the cell membrane.

Several membrane proteins, all of which are bound to the membrane by a glycosyl-phosphatidylinositol (GPI) anchor, are either missing or reduced because of a defect in the synthesis of the GPI anchor resulting from a deficiency of **p**hosphatidyl**i**nositol **g**lucosyltransferase (product of the *PIG-A* gene) due to an acquired mutation in the X-linked *PIG-A* gene. At least two of the membrane proteins affected (decay-accelerating factor or DAF and the membrane inhibitor of reactive lysis or MIRL) are concerned with the modulation of complement activation and, therefore, protection of the cells against inadvertent complement-mediated lysis. The affected cells are thus unusually sensitive to lysis by the terminal complement complex (C5–C9). The essential features of the disease are intravascular haemolysis, recurrent venous thrombosis and pancytopenia. The haemolysis is usually mild and chronic but may be severe and episodic with haemoglobulinuria, which is predominantly nocturnal. The PNH defect may occasionally develop during the course of aplastic anaemia. It may also precede marrow aplasia or develop after recovery from aplasia. Some cases of PNH terminate in acute leukaemia. The diagnosis is usually based on the susceptibility of PNH red cells to undergo lysis when incubated with acidified fresh autologous serum (acidified serum lysis test or the Ham test).

Chronic idiopathic CHAD is treated by keeping the patient warm during the winter and, if necessary, by the use of chlorambucil or cyclophosphamide.

Non-immune haemolytic anaemias

Several of the causes of acquired non-immune haemolytic anaemia are summarized in Table 3.6. Red cells are mechanically damaged when they impact on abnormal surfaces (e.g. cardiac valve prostheses) (Fig. 3.22), or in the case of microangiopathic haemolytic anaemias when they pass across intravascular fibrin strands. Such damage usually results in the presence of red cell fragments in the blood film.

Haemolytic anaemia due to drugs

Any drug that affects essential structural components or functional activities of a red cell is likely to cause a shortening of red cell lifespan. It is not surprising, therefore, that a large number

Table 3.6 Causes of acquired non-immune haemolytic anaemias.

Mechanical trauma to red cells
Abnormalities in the heart and large blood vessels
Aortic valve prostheses (Fig. 3.22), severe aortic valve disease, coarctation of the aorta
Microangiopathic haemolytic anaemia:
Haemolytic uraemic syndrome, thrombotic thrombocytopenic purpura, metastatic malignancy, malignant hypertension, disseminated intravascular coagulation
March haemoglobinuria
Burns
Infections
Clostridium perfringens (welchii), malaria (Figs 3.23 and 3.24), bartonellosis
Drugs,* chemicals and venoms
Oxidant drugs and chemicals, arsine, acute lead poisoning, copper toxicity, venoms of certain spiders and snakes
Hypersplenism

Note: * Some drugs cause haemolysis by immune mechanisms.

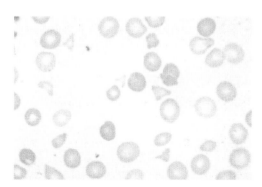

Figure 3.22 Fragmented red cells (schistocytes) in the blood film of a patient with a malfunctioning aortic valve prosthesis.

of drugs have been reported to cause haemolysis. When any haemolytic anaemia is encountered, it is necessary to enquire closely to determine whether there has been any exposure to drugs or chemicals. Some drugs cause haemolysis by non-immune mechanisms and others by immune mechanisms.

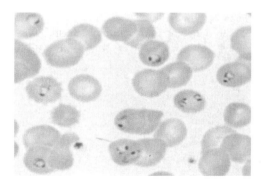

Figure 3.23 Blood film from a patient with *Plasmodium falciparum* malaria showing several parasitized red cells. The ring forms of *Plasmodium falciparum* are smaller and more delicate than those of *Plasmodium vivax* and do not cause enlargement of the parasitized red cells. In falciparum malaria, especially, more than one parasite may be found within a single red cell.

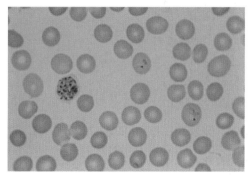

Figure 3.24 Blood film from a patient with *Plasmodium vivax* malaria showing two parasitized red cells each containing a single parasite (ring form or early trophozoite and an ameboid late trophozoite). Another red cell contains a schizont. Some of the parasitized cells were slightly enlarged.

The precise way in which many drugs act on the red cell is not known, but four categories of action can be recognized.

1 Certain chemicals, such as benzene, toluene and saponin, which are fat solvents, act on the red cell membrane and disrupt its lipid components.
2 Certain drugs, such as primaquine, the sulphonamides and phenacetin oxidize and denature Hb and other cell components in people with a deficiency of G6PD or some other red cell enzymes

(p. 32). However, if given in a large enough dose these drugs also affect normal red cells. When given in conventional doses, the two oxidant drugs dapsone and sulphasalazine cause haemolysis in most patients.

3 There are drugs that combine with components on the surface of the red cell and generate complexes that act as antigens. The resulting antibody then reacts with the drug–cell surface complex and brings about red cell destruction. Penicillin, when given in very large doses (more than 6g/day), can occasionally cause a haemolytic anaemia in this way. Certain drugs (e.g. quinidine, quinine, sulphonamides) become antigenic after combining with serum proteins. The antibodies produced form circulating antigen–antibody complexes that become adsorbed onto the red cell surface. The adsorbed antigen–antibody complexes were once thought to activate complement and thereby cause lysis of the affected red cells (the 'innocent bystander' mechanism) but the mechanism of complement activation is now known to be more complex. Such drugs also attach with low affinity to the red cell surface and the drug-dependent antibodies have a specificity not only for the drug but also for red cell membrane antigens.

4 Methyldopa and mefenamic or flufenamic acid trigger the development of an AIHA associated with warm-reactive autoantibodies, perhaps by an effect of the drug on suppressor T-lymphocytes.

Hypersplenism

The term 'hypersplenism' is used to describe the reduction in the lifespan of red cells, granulocytes and platelets that may be found in patients with splenomegaly due to any cause. The cytopenias found in patients with enlarged spleens are also partly caused by increased pooling of blood cells within the spleen and an increased plasma volume; the magnitude of both these effects is proportioned to spleen size. In some haematological diseases in which anaemia is caused by a congenital or acquired defect of the red cell or impaired red cell formation, increasing splenomegaly may result in increasing anaemia by the mechanisms mentioned above.

Chapter 4

Iron Metabolism, Iron Deficiency Anaemia, Other Hypochromic Microcytic Anaemias and Iron Overload

Learning objectives

- To know about the dietary sources, mechanism of absorption, site of storage and method of plasma transportation of iron, and the mechanism and extent of iron loss in men and women.
- To know the causes of iron deficiency at all ages and in both sexes.
- To know the stages of iron deficiency and progression from iron depletion to iron deficiency anaemia.
- To know the mode of presentation of iron deficiency anaemia.
- To know the changes in the morphology of the red cells, in the red cell indices, in the serum levels of iron, transferrin and ferritin, and in the bone marrow iron stores associated with iron deficiency.
- To know how to differentiate between the anaemia due to chronic disorders and that due to iron deficiency.
- To know the principles of treatment of iron deficiency, both by the oral and parenteral routes.
- To know the causes of hypochromic microcytic red cells other than iron deficiency.
- To understand the causes and consequences of iron overload.

Iron deficiency anaemia is the most common type of anaemia throughout the world, affecting about 25% of the world population. Its prevalence in poor countries is considerably higher than in rich

Lecture Notes: Haematology, by NC Hughes-Jones, SN Wickramsinghe, CSR Hatton © 2008 Blackwell Publishing, ISBN: 9781405180504

countries. Iron deficiency anaemia is an important world health problem for three main reasons. Firstly, anaemia in pregnancy (due mainly to iron deficiency) is associated with an increased risk of low birth weight, prematurity and perinatal mortality. Secondly, there is evidence that infants and children with iron deficiency anaemia have impaired psychomotor development and cognitive performance. Thirdly, iron deficient people have a decreased work capacity.

Metabolism of iron

Distribution of iron in the body

Essential iron-containing compounds are found in the plasma and in all cells. Since ionized iron is toxic, virtually all of the iron is present within the haem moiety of a haemoprotein (e.g. haemoglobin (Hb), myoglobin (Mb) and cytochrome) or directly bound to a protein (e.g. transferrin, ferritin and haemosiderin). The total body iron content of a healthy adult varies between 2 and 5 g. About two-thirds of this iron is found in the Hb of red cells; since 1 mL of red cells contains approximately 1 mg of iron, an adult has about 2 g of iron in the red cell mass. About 0.15 g of iron is present in the Mb of muscle cells and in the respiratory enzymes of all cells. Most of the remainder of the iron is stored in the macrophages of the spleen and bone marrow and in both the Kupffer

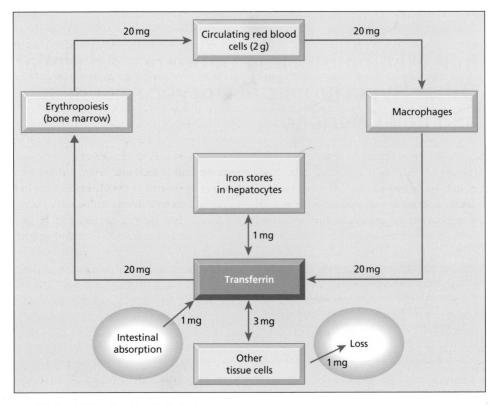

Figure 4.1 The daily kinetics of iron in the body.

and parenchymal cells of the liver. The stores of iron vary from 0 to 1g or more. Storage iron exists in the two forms, ferritin and haemosiderin. Ferritin is water-soluble and is composed of a protein shell that encloses an iron core containing up to 4500 atoms of iron. Haemosiderin is insoluble and is composed of aggregates of ferritin molecules that have partly lost their protein shell. Haemosiderin appears as golden-brown granules in unstained preparations or as blue granules inside macrophages when stained by Perls' acid ferrocyanide method (Prussian Blue reaction). As ferritin is water-soluble, it is leached out during the preparation of histological sections and is not detectable by the Prussian Blue reaction.

Dynamic state of body iron

Iron is continuously circulating through the plasma bound to the protein, transferrin. The major part of this circulating iron is derived from the daily destruction of approximately 20mL of red cells by bone marrow and splenic macrophages and to a lesser extent Kupffer cells, which liberate 20mg of iron (Fig. 4.1). The exit of iron from macrophages is mediated by ferroportin, the same transmembrane protein involved in the exit of iron from enterocytes. There is also a further 5mg of iron carried through the plasma daily. This iron is derived from the iron stores and from absorption in the gastrointestinal tract. Plasma iron is rapidly removed, mainly by erythropoietic tissue in the bone marrow, but part goes to other dividing cells and to the iron stores. The half-time for passage of iron through the circulation depends on the plasma iron concentration and varies between 50 and 110min.

Iron absorption

Iron is present in both vegetables and meat. An average omnivorous diet contains approximately

10–20 mg of iron per day, mostly in ferric–protein and haem–protein complexes (the latter derived from foods of animal origin) but also in inorganic form.

Adults who have normal iron stores absorb approximately 5–10% of their total intake (i.e. they absorb 0.5–2 mg/day). Iron is absorbed mainly in the duodenum. The haem molecule is absorbed best; it is taken up by intestinal epithelial cells within which the iron is split from the porphyrin ring by haem oxygenase. Non-haem iron is less well absorbed as it can be readily bound and made non-absorbable by ligands such as phytate and phosphate that are found in food; its solubilization and absorption is promoted by gastric HCl. Solubilization of non-haem iron is also enhanced by formation of complexes with peptides derived from the digestion of animal protein. Ferric iron must be reduced to the ferrous form before absorption; this is mediated by duodenal cytochrome b located in the apical brush border membrane of the duodenal enterocyte. The ferrous iron is then transported into the enterocyte by the divalent metal transporter, DMT1. Ascorbic acid promotes the absorption of non-haem iron, partly because it is a reducing agent and partly because it forms a molecular complex with it, which is readily absorbed.

Absorption of iron does not remain constant at 5–10% of total intake but is inversely related to the size of iron stores and directly related to the rate of erythropoiesis. When iron intake is in excess of that required for growth and to replenish the daily loss of iron from the body, iron is stored in the liver, spleen and bone marrow. As iron stores increase, the rate of accumulation in the stores decreases, mainly due to a slowing in the rate of absorption. Eventually an equilibrium is reached when iron stores remain constant. On the other hand, when iron stores decrease, the absorptive mechanism is stimulated and the percentage of iron absorbed is increased so that, in iron deficiency, absorption may rise to over 50% of the total intake.

Iron that enters from the gut contents into the epithelial cells is either passed on to the plasma transferrin or remains within the cells and combines with apoferritin to form ferritin. The transfer of iron from the epithelial cells into the plasma is preceded by oxidation to the ferric state by the transmembrane protein hephaestin and mediated by the transmembrane transporter, ferroportin, located in the basolateral membrane of the duodenal enterocyte. It is regulated by unidentified mechanisms that normally respond to iron requirements; the transfer is increased when iron stores are reduced ('stores regulator') or the rate of erythropoiesis is increased ('erythroid regulator'). Iron not transferred to the plasma remains in the epithelial cells until desquamation takes place and the iron is then excreted in the faeces. In pathological states with marked erythroid hyperplasia due to grossly ineffective eythropoiesis, iron absorption is considerably increased in the face of increasing iron stores suggesting that in this situation the 'stores regulator' is subordinate to the 'erythroid regulator.'

Iron loss

There is no specific excretory mechanism for iron. Nevertheless, there is an inevitable daily loss of iron as a result of the continuous exfoliation of gut and skin epithelial cells, all of which have iron-containing enzymes. In adults, this loss is approximately 1 mg/day. The extra loss in women due to menstruation and pregnancy is discussed later (p. 54).

Assessment of iron status

Serum iron and transferrin concentrations and the extent of transferrin saturation

The serum iron is decreased and serum transferrin is frequently increased in iron deficiency (Table 4.1). The transferrin concentration is now readily measured immunochemically. In the past it was measured indirectly by determining the maximum amount of iron that can be bound in serum, that is the total iron-binding capacity (TIBC). In iron deficiency anaemia, the serum transferrin concentration is invariably raised when the Hb concentration falls below 9 g/dL, and is often raised

Table 4.1 Measurements of iron status in people with normal iron stores, individuals with iron depletion without anaemia, and in iron deficiency anaemia.

		Depleted iron stores		
	Normal iron stores	Without reduction of iron supply to tissues	Reduced iron supply to tissues, no anaemia	Iron deficiency anaemia
Serum ferritin (µg/L)	20–300	Usually <20	<20	<20
Transferrin (g/L)	1.7–3.4	Sometimes >3.4	>3.4	>3.4
Serum iron (µmol/L)	10–30	Normal	<10	<10
Transferrin saturation (%)	>16	>16	<16	<16
Hb concentration	Normal	Normal	Within reference range	Below reference range

when the Hb is in the range of 9–11 g/dL. Thus, a raised transferrin concentration is a useful diagnostic criterion, although the finding of raised levels in those taking oral contraceptives reduces its value considerably. The transferrin concentration is frequently reduced below normal in patients with infections, neoplasms and rheumatoid arthritis and thus helps to distinguish anaemia in these diseases from that due to iron deficiency.

An additional useful index is the extent of transferrin saturation, that is the amount of iron bound to transferrin expressed as a percentage of the TIBC (Table 4.1). Values of 16% or lower are usually found when there is an impaired supply of iron to the tissues, as is the case in some individuals with a lack of iron stores and in patients with iron deficiency anaemia. Low values may also be found in the anaemia of chronic disorders.

Serum ferritin levels

Serum ferritin concentration roughly correlates with the amount of tissue-storage iron, when the serum ferritin is below about 4000µg/L. Within this range, a serum level of 100µg/L represents about 1 g of storage iron. Ferritin levels are low in iron deficiency (see Table 4.1). However, there is no single value for ferritin concentration that clearly separates subjects with iron stores from subjects

without, and there is a considerable overlap in ferritin levels between these two groups (Fig. 4.2). In the study illustrated in Fig. 4.2, all women with ferritin levels below 14µg/L were iron deficient; on the other hand, 25% of the iron deficient women had ferritin levels above this value. High serum ferritin levels may be found in the presence of normal or reduced iron stores in acute and chronic infections and malignancy; this results from an increase in ferritin synthesis mediated by macrophage-derived inflammatory cytokines and nitric oxide. High serum ferritin levels are also seen in hepatitis and splenic or bone marrow infarction due to the release of ferritin from these ferritin-rich tissues.

Serum transferrin receptor concentration

The transferrin receptor is present on all cells and iron gains entry by endocytosis following binding of the transferrin–iron complex to the receptor. Serum transferrin receptors are a truncated soluble form of the receptor released into the circulation, mainly by erythroblasts. A deficiency of iron results in an increase in the synthesis of receptors on the erythroblast surface and a 2- to 3-fold increase in serum transferrin receptor concentration; serum levels are not affected by conditions that give rise to the anaemia of chronic disease. Serum transferrin receptor levels also increase in patients with erythroid hyperplasia, independent of iron status.

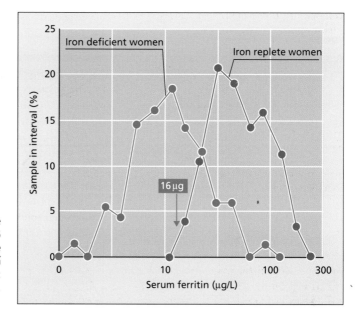

Figure 4.2 The distribution of the serum ferritin concentration in 105 women with stainable iron in the bone marrow (•) and in 69 women with no stainable iron (•). *Source:* From Hallberg *et al.* (1993) *Br. J. Haematol.* **85**, 787–98.

Iron depletion and iron deficiency anaemia

As iron stores are depleted, three phases can be recognized.

1 Depletion of iron stores without diminished iron supply to tissues and without anaemia.
2 Further depletion of iron stores resulting in some reduction of iron supply to tissues. At this stage, transferrin saturation is <16%; serum transferrin receptor concentration is increased due to upregulation of receptors on the erythroblasts; Hb and mean cell volume (MCV), as well as mean cell Hb (MCH), are often within the reference range, but the blood film may contain occasional hypochromic red cells.
3 Continuing depletion of body iron leading to further reduction of iron supply, a fall in Hb concentration, and the picture of iron deficiency anaemia.

Iron depletion without anaemia (phases 1 and 2) is far more common than iron deficiency anaemia.

Prevalence of iron deficiency

Iron deficiency anaemia is the most common haematological abnormality and probably the commonest non-infectious disorder throughout the world. Although often found among the poor due to inadequate dietary intake, it is also prevalent among the affluent. Iron deficiency anaemia (as well as iron depletion without anaemia) appears most frequently during three periods of life: namely, in infants and pre-school children of both sexes, in women during the child-bearing period, and in the elderly. There is a high prevalence of iron depletion without anaemia in adolescents.

Causes of iron deficiency

Iron stores become depleted when the rate of absorption of iron is insufficient to replace iron lost from the body. Inadequate absorption may be due to a low iron content of the diet or to impairment of intestinal absorptive mechanisms. On the other hand, loss of iron through haemorrhage may occur at a greater rate than it can be replaced. The causes of iron deficiency are summarized in Table 4.2.

Causes of iron deficiency related to the gastrointestinal tract

When iron deficiency anaemia occurs in men and postmenopausal women and also in younger

Table 4.2 Causes of iron deficiency.

Reduced iron stores at birth due to prematurity.
Inadequate intake (prolonged breast or bottle feeding without iron supplementation, vegetarian diets, poverty).
Increased requirement (pregnancy and lactation).
Chronic haemorrhage.
Uterine (menorrhagia, metrorrhagia).
Gastrointestinal (e.g. hiatus hernia; oesophageal varices; peptic ulceration; Meckel's diverticulum; colonic diverticulosis, ulcerative colitis, carcinoma of the stomach, colon or rectum, haemorrhoids, hereditary telangiectasia (see p. 148), hookworm infestation*).
Others (e.g. self-inflicted, recurrent haematuria).
Malabsorption (coeliac disease, partial gastrectomy, atrophic gastritis).
Chronic intravascular haemolysis leading to haemoglobinuria and haemosiderinuria (rare).

Note: * This is a very common cause of iron deficiency in tropical countries.

women with gastrointestinal symptoms, occult gastrointestinal blood loss must be considered. Such patients usually require endoscopic and radiological studies of the gut. Bleeding from various lesions in the upper gastrointestinal tract is about 3 times as common as from lesions in the colon.

Partial gastrectomy carried out by the Polya method (common before 1960) is frequently followed by iron deficiency. This is caused by inadequate absorption of iron due to abnormally rapid passage of food through the duodenum. In addition, bleeding from the mucosa of the remnant of the stomach has been observed.

Malabsorption due to coeliac disease is an important cause of iron deficiency and iron deficiency anaemia as is impaired iron absorption due to achlorhydria associated with autoimmune atrophic gastritis. Iron deficiency may also be caused by inadequate dietary intake, especially in those with a restrictive vegetarian diet (e.g. macrobiotic or vegan) as non-haem iron tends to be poorly absorbed (see p. 51).

Causes of iron deficiency in infancy

Two factors predispose to iron deficiency in infancy; namely, inadequate iron stores at birth, and inadequate amounts of iron in the diet. The amount of iron derived from the mother is dependent on her iron status. A child born to an iron deficient mother is about 6 times as likely to develop iron deficiency anaemia compared to a child born to a mother with adequate iron stores. As about half the iron stores are deposited in the last month of fetal life, premature babies may deplete their iron stores before starting on iron-rich solid food. The growing child needs to absorb 0.5–1.0 mg of iron each day during the first year and this cannot be supplied by human milk since it has a low concentration of iron. Infants that are not breast fed should be given an iron-supplemented milk formula. Furthermore, weaning should be introduced between 4 and 6 months to ensure that iron requirements are met.

Causes of iron deficiency in women of child-bearing age

The prevalence of iron deficiency is high in women because of excessive loss of iron through menstruation and loss of iron through child bearing (see below) and lactation.

Iron loss through menstruation

In many women the amount of menstrual blood loss is sufficient to reduce the iron stores rapidly; most women losing more than 60 mL of blood with each period are either iron depleted or have iron deficiency anaemia. The monthly menstrual blood loss in normal women ranges from less than 10 to 180 mL (Fig. 4.3). The diagram also indicates the approximate iron requirements (assuming absorption of 10% of the dietary iron) and it can be seen that women losing 60 mL of blood require about 20 mg of iron in their daily diet, which is about the maximum contained in a normal diet.

Causes of iron deficiency in pregnancy

Haemoglobin concentration falls in pregnancy and normal lower limits have been variously reported to be between 10 and 12 g/dL; the World Health Organization (WHO) has recommended that a

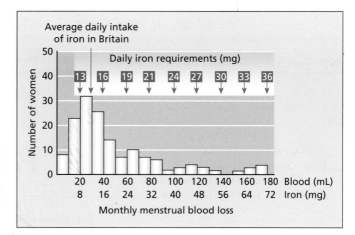

Figure 4.3 Menstrual blood loss in 151 normal women. The daily iron requirements are calculated on the basis that 10% of the iron in the diet is absorbed. *Source*: Jacobs *et al.* (1965) *Postgrad. Med. J.* **41**, 418–24.

lower limit of 11 g/dL should be taken for practical purposes. The main reason for this fall is an increase in plasma volume; red cell mass increases by 200–500 mL but there is an even greater increase in plasma volume resulting in haemodilution. This increase in red cell mass requires an extra 200–500 mg of iron, but this is offset by the fact that there is a reduction in iron loss by approximately the same amount due to amenorrhoea.

The total amount of iron required by the mother during each pregnancy is high, being of the order of 500–700 mg. The fetus requires approximately 250 mg; the rest is lost in the placenta and through hemorrhage — the average blood loss during parturition is of the order of 300 mL. Thus, pregnant women need to absorb, each day, about 2–3 mg more iron than when not pregnant. This is more than can be absorbed from a normal unsupplemented diet, and unless the mother starts pregnancy with more than about 200 mg of storage iron, iron depletion will almost certainly occur. Both iron depletion and iron deficiency anaemia may therefore develop during pregnancy, their prevalence varies in different countries, depending on the iron status of the non-pregnant female population.

Clinical presentation

Symptoms

Iron deficiency anaemia develops slowly, thereby permitting various adaptive mechanisms to operate and compensate for the effects of the developing anaemia (p. 17). Consequently, symptoms caused by the anaemia are usually only seen when Hb falls below about 8 g/dL. These are described on p. 17.

Symptoms attributable to effects of iron deficiency on epithelial tissues or the gastrointestinal tract include a sore mouth, brittle nails, and dysphagia. The combination of postcricoid dysphagia, associated in some cases with a web or stricture, atrophic glossitis and iron deficiency anaemia is known as the Paterson–Kelly or Plummer–Vinson syndrome. The dysphagia, web and anaemia disappear after iron therapy.

Peculiar dietary cravings (pica), for example for soil, clay, chalk or ice, may be found in some cases of iron deficiency anaemia. The ingestion of clay or chalk, which contain substances that form insoluble complexes with non-haem iron in the gut, may be the cause rather than an effect of iron deficiency.

Infants and children with iron deficiency anaemia are not as successful in tests of mental and motor development as their normal counterparts. Treatment with iron has both immediate and long-term beneficial effects.

Signs

The signs of anaemia are listed on p. 17. In addition to these, the following signs resulting from a deficiency of iron in epithelial tissues may be

55

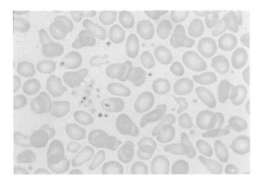

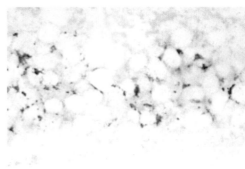

Figure 4.4 Peripheral blood film from a patient with untreated iron deficiency anaemia. Hypochromic microcytes and elongated ('pencil-shaped') poikilocytes are present.

Figure 4.5 Marrow fragment containing normal quantities of storage iron. The haemosiderin stains blue (Perls' acid ferrocyanide stain).

found: redness of the tongue and loss of papillae (glossitis); abnormal nails, either spoon-shaped (koilonychia) or flat; and angular stomatitis. As severe iron deficiency anaemia that has remained untreated for long periods is less common now, these signs of epithelial iron deficiency are less frequently seen today than in the past. The tip of the spleen is palpable in about 10% of cases.

Haematological changes

In patients with depleted iron stores and some reduction of iron supply to the erythron, there may be occasional hypochromic red cells in the blood film at a time when the Hb, MCV and MCH are all within the reference range. However, these values may be below the normal value for that person when iron supply is adequate. As the iron supply becomes progressively reduced, the Hb, MCV and MCH fall progressively. The blood film shows red cells with hypochromia (p. 18), a reduced diameter (microcytosis), and increased variation in size (anisocytosis) and shape (poikilocytosis) (Fig. 4.4). Some poikilocytes are elongated or pencil-shaped. Target cells may also be present. There is a suboptimal increase of the reticulocyte count for the degree of anaemia.

A marrow smear stained by Perls' acid ferrocyanide method shows an absence of stainable iron in the macrophages within the bone marrow

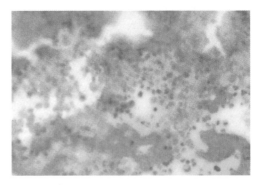

Figure 4.6 Marrow fragment from a patient with iron deficiency anaemia showing an absence of storage iron (Perls' acid ferrocyanide stain).

fragments (Figs 4.5 and 4.6). Erythropoiesis is normoblastic.

Treatment of iron deficiency anaemia

Patients should be treated with 200 mg ferrous sulphate (containing 60 mg of iron) orally, 3 times daily. The minimum response in iron deficient patients is a rise in Hb concentration of 2 g/dL in 3 weeks and most have rises in excess of this. If the patient fails to respond, the following possibilities should be considered:

1 That the patient has not taken the tablets because of gastrointestinal side effects such as pain, diarrhoea or constipation. These adverse

effects may be reduced by taking the tablets with food, decreasing the dose of ferrous sulphate or changing to ferrous gluconate (containing 35 mg of iron in each 300 mg tablet).

2 If the iron deficiency was due to haemorrhage, this may still be operative (e.g. continued bleeding from the gut).

3 That the patient has a severe malabsorption syndrome.

4 That vitamin B_{12} or folate deficiency is also present.

5 That the initial diagnosis was incorrect (e.g. the patient may have thalassaemia trait or anaemia of chronic disorders rather than iron deficiency anaemia).

The purpose of treatment with iron is not only to restore the Hb concentration to normal but also to replenish iron stores. The latter requires continuation of treatment for 4–6 months after the Hb level becomes normal.

Only patients who cannot tolerate any form of iron orally, those in whom substantial blood loss continues and those with a severe malabsorption syndrome should receive iron parenterally. Iron sorbitol (Jectofer) may be given daily by deep intramuscular injection, in a 10-day course. Alternatively, iron sucrose (Venofer) may be given intravenously. Adverse effects, especially of intravenous iron therapy, include anaphylaxis, fever and arthropathy.

Although iron stores are usually absent in pregnancy, there is controversy as to whether all pregnant women should be treated with iron irrespective of their Hb concentration or whether iron should be given only when the Hb falls below an arbitrary value (such as 11 g/dL, p. 16). The argument against treating all pregnant women with iron is that when this is done, haematological investigations may be omitted, so that other causes of anaemia (such as folate deficiency) are missed. Moreover, a considerable proportion of patients do not take the prescribed tablets and do not inform the obstetrician of this. Some are of the opinion that it is safest to estimate the Hb concentration frequently and prescribe iron when required.

> **Key facts**
> *Iron deficiency anaemia*
>
> - Most common form of anaemia.
> - Red cells are hypochromic and microcytic.
> - Serum iron concentration, percentage of transferrin saturation and serum ferritin levels are all low and marrow iron stores are absent.
> - Serum transferrin receptor concentration is increased.
> - Menorrhagia is a common cause in premenopausal women.
> - In men and postmenopausal women, chronic gastrointestinal blood loss should be considered as a cause and, in particular, carcinoma of the stomach and large bowel should be excluded.

Other hypochromic microcytic anaemias

Hypochromic microcytic red cells are formed when there is a substantial impairment of the synthesis of the haem moiety or of the α- or β-globin chains of the Hb molecule. Iron deficiency is the most common cause of these changes; some of the other causes are listed in Table 4.3. Table 4.4 shows the way in which the three most common causes of hypochromia and microcytosis can be distinguished from each other on the basis of the concentrations in the serum of

Table 4.3 Causes of hypochromic and/or microcytic red cells.

Iron deficiency
Anaemia of chronic disorders[a]
Sideroblastic anaemias[a]
Lead poisoning[a]
Heterozygosity and homozygosity for β-thalassaemia[b]
α^+-thalassaemia trait[b,c]
α^0-thalassaemia trait[b]
HbH disease[b]
Heterozygotes and homozygotes for HbE[b,c]
Homozygotes for HbC

Notes: [a] The hypochromia is caused by impaired haem synthesis.
[b] The hypochromia and/or microcytosis is caused by impaired globin chain synthesis.
[c] Some patients have normochromic normocytic red cells.

Table 4.4 Investigations useful in distinguishing between three important causes of hypochromic microcytes.

Investigation	Iron deficiency anaemia	Anaemia of chronic disorders	Thalassaemia trait
Serum iron	Low	Low	Normal
Serum transferrin	Increased or normal	Decreased or normal	Normal
Serum ferritin	Decreased	Normal or increased	Normal
Serum transferrin receptor	Increased	Normal or decreased	Normal or increased
Marrow iron stores	Absent	Normal or increased	Normal or increased

iron, transferrin, ferritin and serum transferrin receptor and the quantity of stainable iron within bone marrow macrophages.

Anaemia of chronic disorders

A common type of anaemia seen in hospital inpatients is that associated with chronic disorders such as chronic infections (e.g. tuberculosis), neoplasia and rheumatoid arthritis. The anaemia is primarily the result of the underproduction of red cells; there is also a mild to moderate reduction in red cell lifespan. The red cells are most often normocytic and normochromic, although in 30–35% of patients they are hypochromic and microcytic. The anaemia usually develops within the first 2 months of the disease and then stabilizes at a fairly constant level.

The pattern of alteration in iron metabolism usually permits the distinction between anaemia of chronic disorder and iron deficiency. In both conditions, the serum iron concentration is low but the two can be distinguished by serum ferritin and transferrin measurements and by serum erythropoietin receptor levels (Table 4.4). Iron deficiency is characterized by low serum ferritin, high transferrin and high serum erythropoietin receptor levels whereas, in contrast, in anaemia of chronic disorders, the ferritin is normal or high, the transferrin frequently low, and the serum transferrin receptor usually normal. In addition, if the MCV is below 70 fL, iron deficiency is much more likely to be present. If the diagnosis from the peripheral blood tests is still in doubt, the presence or absence of storage iron in the marrow can be determined. Characteristically, iron stores are normal or increased in the anaemia of chronic disorders and absent in iron deficiency anaemia.

The pathogenesis of anaemia associated with chronic diseases is complex and is related to the activation of cellular immunity and the release of various inflammatory cytokines such as interleukin (IL)-1, IL-6 and tumour necrosis factor (TNF)-α. Particularly IL-6 and TNF-α induce the synthesis of hepcidin, a circulating peptide, by the liver. This peptide inhibits the absorption of iron in the duodenum and the release of iron from macrophages and consequently reduces the availability of iron for erythroid precursors. Other pathogenetic mechanisms include: (i) suppression of erythropoiesis (including reduced expression of the erythropoietin receptor on erythroblasts) by proinflammatory cytokines such as TNF and IL-1 (produced by activated macrophages) and γ-interferon; (ii) low erythropoietin levels for the degree of anaemia; and (iii) increased erythrophagocytosis by activated macrophages.

Sideroblastic anaemias

The term 'sideroblastic erythropoiesis' is used to describe an abnormal type of red cell production in which a substantial proportion of erythroblasts contain a perinuclear ring of coarse iron-containing granules (Fig. 4.7). These granules are not usually apparent in Romanowsky-stained marrow smears but appear blue in smears stained by Perls' acid ferrocyanide method for haemosiderin. The abnormal cells are described as ring sideroblasts. Ultrastructural studies have shown that the granules within the ring sideroblasts consist of

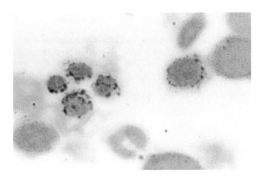

Figure 4.7 Marrow smear from a patient with primary acquired sideroblastic anaemia, stained by the Perls' acid ferrocyanide method (Prussian blue reaction). The erythroblasts contain several coarse (blue–black) iron-containing granules which are often arranged around the nucleus.

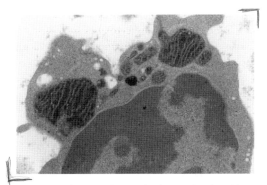

Figure 4.8 Electron micrograph of part of a ring sideroblast showing very electron-dense material between the cristae of enlarged mitochondria.

iron-laden mitochondria; the iron-containing material is deposited in between the mitochondrial cristae (Fig. 4.8). As a result of the mitochondrial damage, a variable proportion of the red cells produced are microcytic and hypochromic.

Sideroblastic erythropoiesis may be found both as an inherited (usually X-linked recessive) and an acquired condition. The common form of X-linked sideroblastic anaemia is caused by mutations in the erythroid-specific δ-aminolaevulinate synthase gene (*ALAS 2* gene). (ALAS is the enzyme catalyzing the first step in haem synthesis.) Pyridoxal phosphate is required both for enzyme activity and enzyme stability and some patients respond to high doses of pyridoxine given orally.

The abnormality occurs as an acquired condition in the myelodysplastic syndrome known as refractory anaemia with ring sideroblasts (primary acquired sideroblastic anaemia) (p. 127), and in occasional patients with chronic myeloproliferative disorders. Acquired sideroblastic anaemia may also be secondary to excessive alcohol consumption, therapy with certain drugs (e.g. isoniazid or chloramphenicol), and lead poisoning.

Iron overload

As the body has no mechanism for actively increasing iron excretion, a progressive increase in total body iron stores occurs in two categories of patients: (i) those who absorb increased quantities of iron over a prolonged period and (ii) those who receive repeated blood transfusions over several years for conditions such as thalassaemia major, aplastic anaemia, and red cell aplasia.

Iron absorption from a normal diet is inappropriately increased from birth in the condition known as hereditary haemochromatosis, which is inherited as an autosomal recessive trait. The gene involved (*HFE*) is located on chromosome 6, close to the HLA-A locus, and most patients have the same point mutation in the gene product (C282Y). The mutation is common in people of Northern European ancestry. Homozygotes usually develop symptoms from tissue damage due to severe iron overload between the ages of 40 and 60 years. There are at least four much rarer forms of hereditary haemochromatosis that are due to mutations in genes other than the *HFE* gene. Iron absorption is also increased in patients with severe erythroid hyperplasia due to peripheral haemolysis or ineffectiveness of erythropoiesis. Some patients in the latter category (e.g. with thalassaemia intermedia or inherited sideroblastic anaemia) may have iron overload even when they have not been transfused to any significant extent.

When the iron stores become greatly increased (Fig. 4.9), the heart, liver, endocrine organs and other tissues undergo progressive damage. Clinicopathological manifestations of severe iron overload

Figure 4.9 Marrow fragment from a chronically transfused patient with aplastic anaemia showing a marked excess of storage iron, compared with the normal amounts shown in Fig. 4.5 (Perls' acid ferrocyanide stain).

include a bronze skin pigmentation, cardiac dysfunction, cirrhosis, diabetes mellitus, testicular atrophy and arthropathy.

The transferrin saturation is increased early during the development of iron overload. The serum ferritin level gives a rough estimate of the extent of iron overload, especially with ferritin values below 4000µg/L, and may be as high as 10,000µg/L in severely affected patients. The diagnosis of iron overload may be confirmed by liver biopsy, which permits both a reliable chemical estimation of the quantity of iron in the tissue and a histological assessment of the distribution of haemosiderin and the extent of tissue damage. In the case of hereditary haemochromatosis, *HFE* genotyping is a valuable diagnostic tool.

Hereditary haemochromatosis is treated by repeated phlebotomy. Iron overload secondary to blood transfusion should be prevented or limited by the administration of the iron chelator desferrioxamine. Patients who are developing iron overload secondary to greatly increased erythropoietic activity should also be treated with desferrioxamine.

Chapter 5

Macrocytosis and Macrocytic Anaemia

Learning objectives

- To understand the relationship between the terms macrocytic, megaloblastic, vitamin B_{12} deficiency and folate deficiency.
- To know the dietary sources, mechanisms of absorption, extent and site of storage, and the mechanism and rate of loss from the body of both B_{12} and folate.
- To be aware of the causes of B_{12} deficiency and of folate deficiency.
- To know the symptoms and signs of B_{12} deficiency referable to the haemopoietic system, central nervous system, peripheral nerves and gastrointestinal tract.
- To understand the principles involved in making the diagnosis of pernicious anaemia from various laboratory investigations.
- To understand the method of differentiation of megaloblastic anaemia due to B_{12} deficiency from that due to folate deficiency.
- To understand the principles of treatment with both B_{12} and folate.
- To know the B_{12}- and folate-independent causes of macrocytosis.

 → red cells (big)

Macrocytosis and macrocytic anaemia may be found in a variety of unrelated diseases. In some conditions associated with macrocytosis, the red cell precursors have a normal morphology

Lecture Notes: Haematology, by NC Hughes-Jones, SN Wickramsinghe, CSR Hatton © 2008 Blackwell Publishing, ISBN: 9781405180504

(i.e. there is normoblastic erythropoiesis) and in others they show morphological abnormalities of the type seen in vitamin B_{12} deficiency caused by pernicious anaemia. Marrows containing such abnormal erythroblasts are described as displaying megaloblastic erythropoiesis. During the investigation of the cause of a macrocytic anaemia it is helpful to determine the type of erythropoiesis by examining stained smears of bone marrow cells obtained by aspiration biopsy. However, a diagnosis can often be made without marrow aspiration.

Megaloblastic erythropoiesis

The causes of megaloblastic erythropoiesis are:

1. A deficiency of vitamin B_{12} or folate.
2. Disturbances of vitamin B_{12} or folate metabolism (e.g. caused by nitrous oxide (N_2O) or methotrexate).
3. Biochemical abnormalities unrelated to vitamin B_{12} or folate (e.g. orotic aciduria; therapy with antipurines).

Megaloblastic erythropoiesis is characterized by abnormal red cell precursors known as megaloblasts, in which cell and nuclear diameters are larger than in normal red cell precursors (normoblasts) and in which the condensed nuclear chromatin is more finely dispersed than in normoblasts of corresponding cytoplasmic maturity (Fig. 5.1). Marrows showing megaloblastic erythropoiesis also

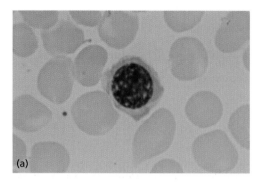
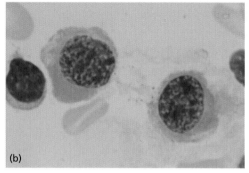

(a)

(b)

Figure 5.1 (a) Early polychromatic normoblast from the marrow of a healthy subject. (b) Early polychromatic megaloblasts from a patient with severe pernicious anaemia. These cells are larger and have a more delicate, sieve-like nucleus containing smaller particles of condensed chromatin than the early polychromatic normoblast.

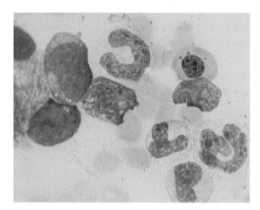

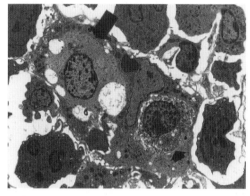

Figure 5.2 Two giant metamyelocytes near a normal-sized metamyelocyte in a marrow smear from a patient with untreated pernicious anaemia. There is also a megaloblast containing Howell–Jolly bodies (i.e. micronuclei).

Figure 5.3 Electron micrograph of a bone marrow macrophage from a patient with severe pernicious anaemia. The cytoplasm of the macrophage contains two ingested megaloblasts (arrowed) at various stages of degradation.

frequently contain giant metamyelocytes. These are about twice the size of normal metamyelocytes and have horseshoe-shaped or long, twisted, ribbon-like nuclei (Fig. 5.2).

Megaloblasts suffer from a gross disturbance of cell proliferation, and many of the more mature megaloblasts are ingested and degraded by bone marrow macrophages (Fig. 5.3). Thus, despite the fact that megaloblastic marrows show erythroid hyperplasia, this increased ineffectiveness of erythropoiesis (p. 11) results in the rate of delivery of new red cells into the circulation being suboptimal for the degree of anaemia. Many of the

giant metamyelocytes are also destroyed within the marrow (ineffective granulocytopoiesis).

Megaloblastic changes occur when DNA synthesis is disordered, but the detailed biochemical basis of the morphological abnormality remains uncertain. The ways in which B_{12} and folate deficiency may impair DNA synthesis are discussed later (pp. 63 and 73).

In B_{12} and folate deficiency, megaloblastic changes are not confined to bone marrow cells; the characteristic nuclear abnormality is found in a variety of epithelial cells, including those of the buccal and nasal mucosa, tongue, urinary tract, jejunum, vagina and cervix uteri.

Blood picture in patients with megaloblastic haemopoiesis

Characteristically, there is a high mean cell volume (MCV) associated with varying degrees of anaemia. Patients diagnosed early have a high MCV without anaemia. However, even in these, the haemoglobin (Hb) level may rise following the correction of the underlying defect indicating that their Hb at presentation, although within the reference range, was below their own normal value. The absolute reticulocyte count is variable, being either reduced, normal, or slightly increased. Any increase is much less than that seen in an individual with normally functioning bone marrow and a similar degree of anaemia. Red cell lifespan is slightly decreased. However, the anaemia is mainly due to the ineffectiveness of megaloblastic erythropoiesis. The blood films of patients with megaloblastic erythropoiesis contain macrocytes, some of which are oval in shape (Fig. 5.4). The red cells also show anisocytosis and poikilocytosis, particularly in moderately and severely anaemic cases. Macrocytic anaemias caused by megaloblastic haemopoiesis are referred to as megaloblastic anaemias.

In patients with B_{12}- or folate-related megaloblastic haemopoiesis, the circulating neutrophil granulocytes frequently show hypersegmentation of their nuclei (Fig. 5.4). Under normal circumstances, 3% or less of neutrophil granulocytes have five or more nuclear segments, but in B_{12} or folic acid deficiency more than 3% are hyper-

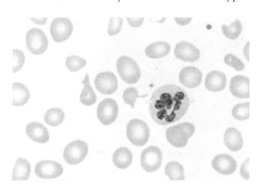

Figure 5.4 Blood film from a patient with pernicious anaemia showing oval macrocytes, other poikilocytes and a hypersegmented neutrophil.

segmented and there may even be occasional cells with 8–10 segments. Hypersegmentation is not diagnostic of B_{12} or folate deficiency; it may also occur in anaemia due to iron deficiency and in renal failure, even when B_{12} and folate stores are adequate. Hypersegmented neutrophil polymorphs are not derived from giant metamyelocytes but from normal-looking metamyelocytes. When the megaloblastic changes caused by B_{12} or folate deficiency are severe, there may be neutropenia and thrombocytopenia (due to ineffective granulocytopoiesis and thrombocytopoiesis).

Megaloblastic anaemias (macrocytic anaemias with megaloblastic erythropoiesis)

Vitamin B_{12} deficiency

Biochemistry

The B_{12} molecule is composed of: (i) a planar corrin nucleus made up of four pyrrole rings (A–D, Fig. 5.5); (ii) the ribonucleotide of 5,6-dimethylbenzimidazole; and (iii) a cobalt atom situated at the centre of the corrin nucleus which is coordinately bonded to the four pyrrole rings, one of the nitrogen atoms of the ribonucleotide and to an organic group (Fig. 5.5). In the two biologically active forms of vitamin B_{12}, namely methylcobalamin and adenosylcobalamin, the organic group bound to the cobalt atom is methyl and adenosyl, respectively.

The biochemical mechanisms underlying the anaemia and neuropathy of B_{12} deficiency are still uncertain. However, both the anaemia and neuropathy may be caused by an impairment of one of the two reactions known to require vitamin B_{12} in man, namely the methylation of homocysteine to methionine by homocysteine methyltransferase, which is dependent both on 5-methyltetrahydrofolate (p. 73) and methylcobalamin.

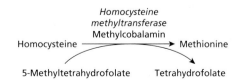

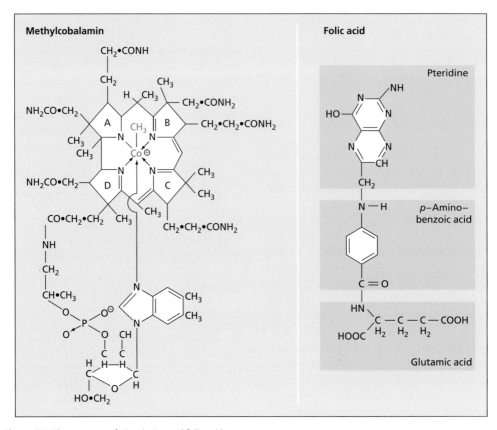

Figure 5.5 The structure of vitamin B_{12} and folic acid.

Since the 5-methyltetrahydrofolate serves as the methyl donor, failure of this reaction results not only in impaired methionine synthesis but also in the accumulation of 5-methyltetrahydrofolate and homocysteine, with increased concentrations of homocysteine in the serum. Impairment of the homocysteine methyltransferase reaction eventually leads to a reduction in the availability of 5,10-methylenetetrahydrofolate for the methylation of deoxyuridine monophosphate (dUMP) to

It has been proposed that impairment of the homocysteine methyltransferase reaction results in reduced levels of 5,10-methylenetetrahydrofolate by the trapping of intracellular folates in the form of 5-methyltetrahydrofolate, which cannot be converted to 5,10-methylenetetrahydrofolate (methylfolate trap hypothesis). However, recent data suggest that the important consequence of the impairment of the homocysteine methyltransferase reaction is not the intracellular accumulation of 5-methyltetrahydrofolate but the failure of methionine synthesis, which in turn results in the reduced synthesis of S-adenosylmethionine and, consequently, a decreased supply of active formate required for the synthesis of 5,10-methylenetetrahydrofolate (formate starvation hypothesis).

The second of the two reactions known to require B_{12} in humans is the adenosylcobalamin-dependent conversion of methylmalonyl CoA to succinyl CoA by the enzyme methylmalonyl CoA mutase.

The involvement of B_{12} in this reaction explains the finding of raised serum methylmalonic acid concentrations in B_{12} deficiency.

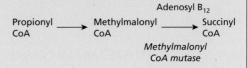

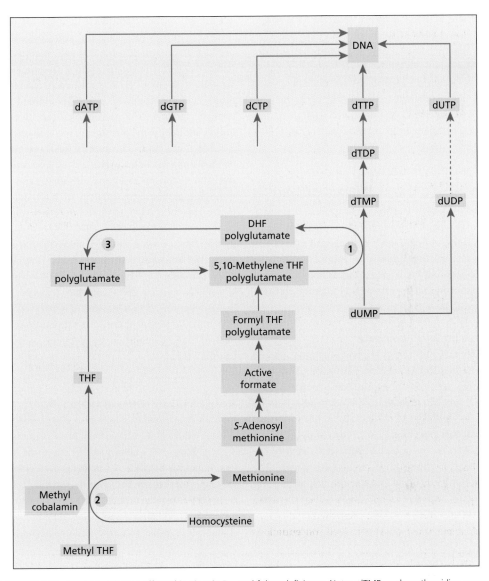

Figure 5.6 Biochemical pathways affected in vitamin B_{12} and folate deficiency. *Notes*: dTMP — deoxythymidine monophosphate; dTTP — deoxythymidine triphosphate; dUMP — deoxyuridine monophosphate; dUTP — deoxyuridine triphosphate; THF — tetrahydrofolate. Enzymes: 1, thymidylate synthase; 2, homocysteine methyltransferase (methionine synthase); 3, dihydrofolate reductase.

thymidine monophosphate and, consequently, to reduced synthesis of thymidine triphosphate (Fig. 5.6). This in turn causes: (a) the slowing of DNA strand elongation due to an inadequate supply of thymidine triphosphate for DNA synthesis; (b) the accumulation of dUMP within the cell and its phosphorylation to deoxyuridine triphosphate (dUTP); and (c) misincorporation into DNA of uracil (from dUTP) in lieu of thymine (Fig. 5.6). Although there is little doubt that DNA synthesis is impaired in B_{12} deficiency, the critical defect underlying the megaloblastic change remains unclear.

There is some evidence that the neuropathy associated with B_{12} deficiency may be caused by hypomethylation of nervous system proteins due to the reduced availability of *S*-adenosylmethionine. Whether impairment of the adenosylcobalamin-dependent conversion of methylmalonyl CoA to succinyl CoA is also involved in the pathogenesis of the neuropathy is controversial.

Vitamin B_{12} in the diet

Vitamin B_{12} is produced entirely by bacteria and none is present in plants. Herbivores obtain vitamin B_{12} mainly as a result of synthesis by bacteria in their rumen; other animals and man obtain it by eating food of animal origin. The average amount of B_{12} in a mixed diet is about $5\,\mu g/day$. The nutritional aspects of this vitamin are summarized in Table 5.1.

Mechanism of absorption

Vitamin B_{12} in food is largely protein-bound and is released from its bound state within the stomach by the action of pepsin. Most of the released B_{12} binds immediately to R-binder (a B_{12}-binding protein found in saliva and gastric juice). The B_{12} is released from the B_{12}-R-binder complex in the jejunum by the action of pancreatic trypsin; the released B_{12} then binds to intrinsic factor. The function of intrinsic factor is to transport B_{12} into the epithelial cells of the distal half of the small intestine.

Intrinsic factor is produced in the body and fundus of the stomach by the same cells that produce hydrochloric acid, namely, the gastric parietal cells. It is a glycoprotein with a molecular weight of about $57\,kDa$ and each molecule binds one molecule of B_{12}. The amount of intrinsic factor in the gastric juice can be estimated indirectly by measuring the amount of B_{12} that it can bind. The average basal secretion of 3000 units per hour increases 3- to 5-fold after the administration of stimulants such as histamine and gastrin. The quantity of B_{12} required to be absorbed daily to maintain body stores is about 1–$3\,\mu g$, and only 1000–3000 units of intrinsic factor are necessary for its absorption. Thus, the amount of intrinsic factor produced daily (probably of the order of 50,000 units) is considerably in excess of that required for B_{12} absorption. The minimum quantity of B_{12} that must be absorbed daily to maintain health (rather than to maintain body stores) may be less than $0.5\,\mu g$.

Storage and rate of loss of vitamin B_{12}

Vitamin B_{12} is mainly stored in the liver and the average healthy adult has a total body content of 3–$5\,mg$. Loss of B_{12} takes place in the urine and faeces mainly through desquamation of epithelial cells and through excretion in the bile. There is an enterohepatic circulation of B_{12}; 3–$6\,\mu g$ is excreted per day into the intestine, mainly in the

Table 5.1 Key features of vitamin B_{12} and folate nutrition and absorption.

	Vitamin B_{12}	Folate
Dietary sources	Only foods of animal origin, especially liver	Most foods, especially liver, green vegetables and yeast; destroyed by cooking
Average daily intake[a]	$5\,\mu g$	$400\,\mu g$
Minimum daily requirement[a]	1–$3\,\mu g$	100–$200\,\mu g$[b]
Body stores[a]	3–$5\,mg$, mainly in the liver	8–$20\,mg$, mainly in the liver
Time to develop deficiency in the absence of intake or absorption[a]	Anaemia in 2–10 years	Macrocytosis in 5 months
Requirements for absorption	Intrinsic factor secreted by gastric parietal cells	Conversion of polyglutamates to monoglutamates by intestinal folate conjugase
Site of absorption	Terminal ileum	Duodenum and jejunum

Notes: [a]In adults. [b]Higher during pregnancy and lactation.

bile, and most of this (except about 1 µg) is normally reabsorbed in the terminal ileum.

The rate of loss of B_{12} is approximately 0.05–0.1% of the body content each day. There is therefore a delay of 2 years or more between the appearance of a lesion leading to impaired absorption of B_{12} and the reduction of the B_{12} store to a level (possibly about 300–500 µg) that causes megaloblastic anaemia. For instance, following the abrupt cessation of B_{12} absorption as a consequence of total gastrectomy, it takes about 2–10 years before megaloblastic anaemia develops.

Vitamin B_{12} neuropathy

Patients with vitamin B_{12} deficiency due to any cause may develop degenerative changes in the nervous system. The pathological changes are often considered under three headings:

1 Peripheral neuropathy.
2 Subacute combined degeneration of the cord.
3 Focal demyelinization of the white matter of the brain.

In subacute combined degeneration of the cord there is patchy degeneration of the posterior and lateral columns which is most marked in (but not confined to) the lower cervical and upper thoracic segments (Fig. 5.7). Histologically, the degenerating areas contain empty spaces that are surrounded by myelin-laden macrophages. The term 'subacute combined degeneration' of the cord is, however, misleading since the onset of symptoms is usually insidious and not subacute, lesions of the posterior and lateral columns can occur alone and are not necessarily combined, and the syndrome frequently includes lesions of the peripheral nerves or cerebral hemispheres as well as the spinal cord.

Symptoms and signs usually affect the lower limbs first and are symmetrical. The commonest symptoms are paraesthesia in the extremities, ataxia of gait and muscle weakness. Others include poor vision, orthostatic dizziness, stiffness of the limbs, impotence and impairment of bladder and rectal control. Some impairment of memory, irritability, mild depression, apathy and fluctuations

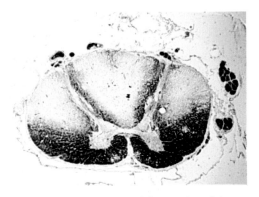

Figure 5.7 Subacute combined degeneration of the cervical spinal cord. The posterior and lateral columns show demyelination and therefore appear pale (Weigert–Pal method for myelin). *Source*: Reproduced with permission from Dr. R.O. Barnard.

of mood are relatively common but serious psychiatric symptoms (e.g. stupor, hallucinations, paranoia, severe depression and manic psychosis) are uncommon. However, occasional patients have been rescued from psychiatric institutions and restored to health by B_{12} injections. Blindness due to optic atrophy has been reported but is rare.

On the basis of a clinical examination of the nervous system, it is sometimes difficult to distinguish between peripheral neuritis and posterior column involvement, since in both conditions tendon reflexes and vibrational and positional sense may be reduced, and ataxia may be present. However, hyperalgesia of calf muscles favours peripheral neuritis, whereas a disproportionate reduction in positional and vibrational sense compared to touch and pinprick favours involvement of the lateral columns. An extensor plantar response indicates pyramidal tract involvement. Individual patients vary in the extent to which lesions in the posterior columns, lateral columns or peripheral nerves dominate the neurological syndrome. Spinal cord lesions may occur in the absence of peripheral neuritis and vice versa. Nerve conduction studies and MR1 scans of the spinal cord are important investigations.

The severity of neurological abnormality correlates inversely with the haematocrit. Neurological involvement may occur without anaemia although the bone marrow usually shows mild megaloblastic changes.

Causes of vitamin B$_{12}$ deficiency

These are summarized in Table 5.2. The two most common causes of vitamin B$_{12}$ deficiency are pernicious anaemia and veganism.

Inadequate intake

Veganism

Vitamin B$_{12}$ deficiency resulting solely from a very low B$_{12}$ content in the diet only occurs in strict vegetarians who eat no animal protein at all (vegans). Although there is no B$_{12}$ in plants, the vegan diet probably contains some B$_{12}$ as a result of bacterial contamination of water and vegetables and bacterial fermentation of bruised vegetables. Low serum B$_{12}$ levels are found in over 50% of vegans. However, most vegans with low serum B$_{12}$ levels are healthy and do not show anaemia or macrocytosis; only a minority suffer from megaloblastic anaemia or B$_{12}$ neuropathy. This results from the presence of very small amounts of B$_{12}$ in the diet and an intact enterohepatic circulation of B$_{12}$ (p. 66).

Inadequate secretion of intrinsic factor

Pernicious anaemia

Pernicious anaemia is a disorder in which the absorption of B$_{12}$ is greatly impaired due to a marked reduction of intrinsic factor secretion secondary to severe atrophic gastritis or gastric atrophy. One of the first descriptions of this condition was by Thomas Addison of Guy's Hospital, London, in 1849, and the disease is therefore sometimes referred to as Addisonian pernicious anaemia. It appears to have a genetically determined autoimmune basis.

Genetic factors and autoimmune processes
About 20% of patients have a relative with pernicious anaemia, indicating that genetic factors may predispose to the development of gastric atrophy in adult life. Furthermore, 10% of patients with pernicious anaemia have clinical or subclinical autoimmune thyroid disease suggesting that

Table 5.2 Mechanisms and causes of vitamin B$_{12}$ deficiency.

Inadequate intake
Veganism, lactovegetarianism (some cases)

Inadequate secretion of intrinsic factor
Pernicious anaemia
Total or partial gastrectomy
Congenital intrinsic factor deficiency (rare)

Inadequate release of B$_{12}$ from food
Partial gastrectomy, vagotomy, gastritis, acid-suppressing drugs, alcohol abuse

Diversion of dietary B$_{12}$
Abnormal intestinal bacterial flora multiple jejunal diverticula, small intestinal strictures, stagnant intestinal loops
Diphyllobothrium latum

Malabsorption
Crohn's disease, ileal resection, chronic tropical sprue, congenital selective B$_{12}$ malabsorption with proteinuria (Imerslund–Gräsbeck syndrome)

---

the gastric atrophy has an autoimmune basis. Antibodies against gastric parietal cells are found in the serum in about 85% of patients with pernicious anaemia; these are directed against the α- and β-subunits of the proton pump (H$^+$, K$^+$ ATPase) of the gastric parietal cell. Antibodies against intrinsic factor are found in the serum of about 55% of patients and in the gastric juice of about 60%. However, the fact that antibodies cannot be detected in all cases, combined with the observation that a few patients with thyroid disorders have anti-intrinsic factor antibodies in their serum but do not have B$_{12}$ deficiency, suggest that these antibodies are not the primary cause of the gastric atrophy and the resulting failure of intrinsic factor secretion. They may instead be a consequence of the damage to the gastric mucosa. It is possible, on the other hand, that the gastric atrophy is the result of cell-mediated immune reactions against parietal and other gastric cells as is the case in a murine model of autoimmune chronic atrophic gastritis.

Gastric lesion
All cases of pernicious anaemia have a gastric lesion, varying from severe atrophic gastritis to

gastric atrophy. The basal secretion of intrinsic factor is reduced to only 0–200 units per hour and is unaffected by stimulants such as histamine. Vitamin B_{12} deficiency develops and leads to megaloblastic anaemia or neurological damage, or both. As both intrinsic factor and hydrochloric acid are produced by the same cell (i.e. the parietal cell), histamine-fast and pentagastrin-fast achlorhydria is an invariable accompaniment of pernicious anaemia and the diagnosis cannot be made if appreciable quantities of hydrochloric acid are found to be secreted. The pH of resting gastric juice in pernicious anaemia is between 6 and 8 and after maximal stimulation with histamine or pentagastrin it does not fall by more than 0.5 pH units. However, not all individuals with gastric atrophy or achlorhydria have pernicious anaemia, presumably because many individuals with these abnormalities continue to secrete the small quantities of intrinsic factor required for the absorption of adequate amounts of B_{12}.

Tissues affected by B_{12} deficiency

Pernicious anaemia should not be regarded merely as a condition in which there is a deficient production of red cells and damage to the nervous system, but rather as a vitamin deficiency disease affecting many cell types in the body, including all dividing cells. Symptoms and signs are referable not only to the blood and neural tissue (brain, spinal cord, peripheral nerves), but also to the gastrointestinal tract (from the tongue down to the colon), skin and other tissues and organs (e.g. ovary and testis). Severe anaemia may aggravate coexisting cardiac disease.

Clinical features

Pernicious anaemia is common in people of northern European extraction but also occurs in Africans, Asians, Chinese and other races. According to the old literature (published at a time when mild B_{12} deficiency could not be easily diagnosed), the prevalence of this disease in England is about one per 1000 of the population. Only 10% of cases are diagnosed under 40 years of age and the prevalence increases with age, reaching about 0.5–1% over the age of 70 years. However, a recent

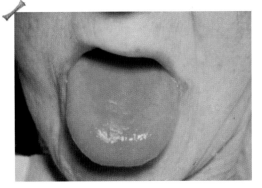

Figure 5.8 Glossitis in a woman with severe pernicious anaemia.

study from California suggests that the prevalence of mild B_{12} deficiency due to undiagnosed pernicious anaemia in people aged 60 years and over is as high as 1.4–4.3%. Females are 1.5 times more frequently affected than males.

Symptoms develop slowly. Common presenting symptoms are tiredness and weakness, dyspnoea, paraesthesia, a sore tongue, vague gastrointestinal disturbance (anorexia, nausea, vomiting, dyspepsia, constipation or diarrhoea) and loss of weight. Other symptoms include subfertility and, rarely, hyperpigmentation of the skin of the hands. Various neurological and psychiatric symptoms may develop in a proportion of cases, due to a B_{12} neuropathy (p. 67). Apart from pallor, the most frequent sign is atrophic glossitis. Commonly, some degree of papillary atrophy of the tongue is seen as an unusual smoothness at the edges, but this sometimes spreads over the entire dorsal surface (Fig. 5.8). Fever may be present when the anaemia is severe. The spleen is palpable in some cases. Autoimmune disorders such as autoimmune thyroid diseases, vitiligo, hypoparathyroidism and hypofunction of the adrenal glands occur with increased frequency in patients and their relatives. In pernicious anaemia, there is an increased incidence of gastric carcinoid tumours but these are usually relatively benign. Male patients have an increased incidence of gastric carcinoma.

Haematological and biochemical changes

The haematological picture is that seen in any B_{12}- or folate-related megaloblastic anaemia (p. 63).

The Hb level may be within the reference range in patients diagnosed early but decreases progressively as the degree of deficiency increases. The blood count shows a high MCV provided that the pernicious anaemia is not complicated by coexisting iron deficiency or thalassaemia trait or is not diagnosed very early. The marrow is hypercellular and in severely anaemic patients virtually all of the fat cells of the marrow are replaced by haemopoietic cells. Haemopoiesis is megaloblastic in type and giant metamyelocytes may be present (p. 62).

There may be a slight increase in the serum bilirubin level and an increase in serum lactate dehydrogenase; these changes result mainly from the intramedullary destruction of erythroblasts and partly from a mild degree of peripheral haemolysis. The level of B_{12} in the serum is virtually always reduced. However, low serum B_{12} levels should be considered as presumptive rather than definitive evidence of B_{12} deficiency, since they are also found in the absence of any other evidence of B_{12} deficiency, in one-third of folate-deficient patients and in some healthy pregnant women. About 60% of patients with pernicious anaemia have low red cell folate levels and the remainder have normal levels. The concentrations of both methylmalonic acid and homocysteine in the serum are raised in virtually all patients.

Diagnosis

In order to establish the diagnosis of pernicious anaemia, it is necessary to demonstrate either a marked reduction or the absence of intrinsic factor in gastric juice (see Table 5.3). This is usually done indirectly by performing a Schilling test. This test measures the ability of an individual to absorb orally administered cyanocobalamin. It involves giving 1 μg of ^{57}Co-cyanocobalamin by mouth and, at the same time, 1 mg of non-radioactive cyanocobalamin intramuscularly. The urine passed over the next 24 h is collected and its radioactivity determined. The large intramuscular dose of non-radioactive B_{12} saturates the B_{12}-binding proteins in the plasma and thus causes a substantial proportion of any absorbed ^{57}Co-B_{12} to be excreted in the urine. B_{12} absorption is considered to be impaired when the urinary excretion of ^{57}Co-B_{12} over the 24 h is less than 11% of the dose given by mouth. In pernicious anaemia it is often below 5%. If the test is abnormal it should be repeated giving both intrinsic factor and ^{57}Co-B_{12} by mouth (part 2 of the Schilling test); if the low B_{12} absorption in the patient is the result of intrinsic factor deficiency, then the absorption will be improved (but not restored to normal). In the DICOPAC test, the two parts of the Schilling test are performed simultaneously by using both

Table 5.3 Tests useful in establishing the diagnosis and cause of vitamin B_{12} deficiency.

Investigation	Findings
Dietary assessment	No intake of animal protein in vegans
Blood count	High MCV*
Blood film	Oval macrocytes,* hypersegmentation of neutrophil granulocytes*
Bone marrow aspiration	Megaloblasts,* giant metamyelocytes*
Serum vitamin B_{12}	Low (also low in one-third of folate-deficient patients)
Red cell folate	Normal or low
Serum methylmalonic acid	Raised
Schilling test for B_{12} absorption	Abnormal in pernicious anaemia, diseases of the terminal ileum and in the 'stagnant loop syndrome'. Abnormality improves when the test is performed with intrinsic factor only in pernicious anaemia
Barium meal and follow through	Demonstrates various lesions of the small intestine in the 'stagnant loop syndrome' and in diseases of the terminal ileum
Assay of intrinsic factor in gastric juice	Very low or absent in pernicious anaemia

Note: * Also found in folate deficiency.

Co^{57}- and Co^{58}- labelled B_{12}, one attached to intrinsic factor.

Intrinsic factor antibodies are present in the serum in 50–60% of cases of pernicious anaemia. Their presence is highly specific for this disorder and if found the diagnosis can be made without doing a Schilling test.

Treatment

Patients with pernicious anaemia may be initially treated with 1 mg hydroxocobalamin intramuscularly every 2–3 weeks over a period of 3 months to replenish body stores. Maintenance therapy with injections of 1 mg hydroxocobalamin every 3 months should be continued for the rest of their lives. It is customary to start treating patients with serious neurological symptoms with 1 mg hydroxocobalamin twice a week rather than every 2–3 weeks even though there is no evidence that more frequent injections are required for the treatment of neuropathy than of anaemia. Complicating infections and congestive cardiac failure should be treated promptly. Blood transfusion should be avoided whenever possible as this may precipitate or aggravate cardiac failure. If transfusion is necessary in severely anaemic patients, this should be done cautiously under cover of diuretics, administering no more than 1–2 units of packed red cells slowly over 24 h. Some clinicians prefer to perform a 1- to 2-unit partial exchange transfusion. A number of patients with severe pernicious anaemia die suddenly, presumably of cardiac arrhythmias, shortly after the start of B_{12} therapy and this has been attributed to a fall in serum potassium consequent on a movement of potassium into cells in response to therapy with B_{12}. Patients with severe pernicious anaemia should therefore be started on oral potassium supplements at the same time as the B_{12}; the potassium should be continued for 10 days. If the cause of a severe megaloblastic anaemia is uncertain at presentation, as is often the case, treatment should be started with both hydroxocobalamin intramuscularly and folic acid orally. It must be emphasized that B_{12} deficiency should not be treated for a prolonged period with folic acid alone since, although the anaemia

> **Key facts**
> *Pernicious anaemia*
>
> - B_{12} absorption is reduced due to marked impairment of intrinsic factor secretion secondary to autoimmune severe atrophic gastritis/gastric atrophy.
> - Several patients give a family history of a relative with pernicious anaemia or other autoimmune disorder, particularly hypothyroidism.
> - Prevalence increases with age; affects about 1% of individuals over 60 years.
> - Presents with (a) macrocytic anaemia with megaloblastic haemopoiesis; and/or (b) B_{12} neuropathy (peripheral neuritis, subacute combined degeneration of the cord).
> - Serum B_{12} level is low and part 1 of the Schilling test shows impaired B_{12} absorption.
> - Some patients have intrinsic factor antibodies and these are virtually specific for pernicious anaemia.
> - Respond to parenteral hydroxocobalamin.

usually responds, neurological lesions do not and may rapidly progress.

Response to hydroxocobalamin is rapid. There is an increase in mental acuity and a sense of well-being within 24–48 h. The reticulocyte response peaks at about 5–7 days and, after the first week, the Hb rises by about 1 g/week (Fig. 5.9). Neurological symptoms of recent onset (less than about 3 months duration) show marked improvement and may even disappear over the first 6–12 months of therapy. More long-standing symptoms improve to a lesser extent. Psychiatric symptoms of recent onset often disappear rapidly and completely.

Total or partial gastrectomy

Megaloblastic anaemia due to B_{12} deficiency is an invariable result of total gastrectomy and develops 2–10 years after the operation, this being the time taken to exhaust the B_{12} stores present preoperatively. Some cases develop B_{12} neuropathy. Parenteral B_{12} therapy should be commenced shortly after the gastrectomy. Anaemia resulting from B_{12} deficiency and, occasionally, subacute combined degeneration of the cord may also develop in 5% of cases subjected to partial

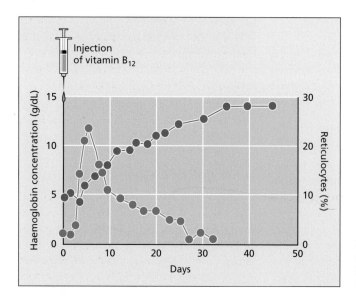

Figure 5.9 Response of a patient with pernicious anaemia to vitamin B_{12} administration: (●) Hb concentration; (●) reticulocyte percentage.

gastrectomy but usually not before 5 years have elapsed. In some cases this is due to the removal of most of the intrinsic factor-producing area of the stomach and atrophy of the remaining mucosa leading to deficiency of intrinsic factor secretion. In other cases the absorption of crystalline B_{12} in the Schilling test is normal and the B_{12} deficiency is caused not by intrinsic factor deficiency, but by a failure to release B_{12} from food (see below). The incidence of deficiency after partial gastrectomy is sufficiently high to warrant routine periodic examination of the blood.

Inadequate release of vitamin B_{12} from food

Some patients who have undergone vagotomy or partial gastrectomy develop B_{12} deficiency due to impaired release of B_{12} from food as a consequence of a reduced secretion of hydrochloric acid and pepsin. There is increasing evidence that unexplained low serum B_{12} levels in patients who have not been subjected to vagotomy or gastric surgery may, in about 45% of cases, also result from inadequate release of B_{12} from food. The pathogenesis of the gastric dysfunction in such cases is currently under investigation and includes the use of acid-suppressing drugs such as cimetidine, ranitidine and omeprazole, non-specific or *Helicobacter pylori*

gastritis and alcohol abuse. Patients may be treated with either oral or parenteral B_{12}.

Diversion of dietary vitamin B_{12}

Abnormal intestinal bacterial flora ('stagnant loop syndrome')

Macrocytic anaemia often arises in patients who have anatomical abnormalities of the small gut (blind loops, fistulae, diverticulosis, anastomoses) which lead to stasis and bacterial overgrowth. Many strains of bacteria found in stagnant small intestinal loops can take up B_{12} and convert it to inactive cobamides, leaving none for absorption by the patient. Folic acid is not affected in this way; in fact folic acid may be produced by these bacteria and therefore red cell folate levels may be high. Patients with this condition give an abnormal result with the Schilling test for B_{12} absorption (both without and with intrinsic factor); the abnormality is corrected after therapy with broad-spectrum antibiotics.

Infestation with the fish tapeworm

Diversion of B_{12} in the gut can occur due to successful competition by the fish tapeworm, *Diphyllobothrium latum*, which was common in Finland, but is now becoming rare.

Malabsorption

Malabsorption of B_{12} due to disease of the terminal ileum may be seen in coeliac disease and regional ileitis, and is almost invariable in chronic tropical sprue. In the latter, B_{12} deficiency is often combined with folate deficiency. Reduced absorption of B_{12} also occurs after resection of the terminal ileum. The Schilling test gives an abnormal result both without and with intrinsic factor.

Diagnosis of vitamin B_{12} deficiency

The investigations that may be of diagnostic value in a patient suspected of suffering from B_{12} deficiency are given in Table 5.3; some of these are discussed in more detail in the preceding sections. It is occasionally difficult to reliably diagnose B_{12} deficiency in patients who may have a deficiency of both B_{12} and folate (i.e. have low concentrations of both serum B_{12} and red cell folate; pp. 70 and 75). In these cases, it is useful to investigate the haematological response to daily injections of $2\mu g$ hydroxocobalamin (i.e. physiological doses of B_{12}) since a response would only occur if there is a deficiency of B_{12}. Commonly, such patients are not investigated in this way but treated with both B_{12} and folate.

Folate deficiency

Biochemistry

Folic acid (pteroylmonoglutamic acid) is composed of three portions: a pteridine nucleus, *p*-aminobenzoic acid and glutamic acid (see Fig. 5.5). This compound is not biochemically active until it is reduced first to dihydrofolic acid and then to tetrahydrofolic acid. In addition, naturally occurring forms of folate contain a single carbon unit in various states of reduction (e.g. methyl, formyl, methylene). Whereas the folate present in the serum is 5-methyltetrahydrofolate monoglutamate, intracellular folates are pteroylpolyglutamates with three to seven glutamic acid residues joined together. The active forms of folate function as coenzymes in the transfer of single carbon units in: (i) amino acid metabolism and (ii) the synthesis of purines and pyrimidines required for DNA and RNA synthesis. In particular, 5,10-methylenetetrahydrofolate is required for the methylation of deoxyuridylate to thymidylate, and an impairment of this reaction may be one of the biochemical abnormalities underlying the altered DNA synthesis and the megaloblastic change in folate deficiency (see p. 64).

Folates in the diet

Folates are found in foods of both animal and plant origin. An average Western diet contains about $400\mu g$ of folate daily. The folate content of food is markedly affected by cooking as folates are rapidly destroyed by heat. About 80% of an oral dose of $200\mu g$ pteroylglutamic acid is absorbed; the percentage absorption of polyglutamates is somewhat lower. In an adult, the minimum quantity of folate required to be absorbed daily is about $100–200\mu g$. The requirement is greater during pregnancy and lactation. The nutritional aspects of folate are compared with those of B_{12} in Table 5.1.

Absorption

This takes place mainly in the duodenum and jejunum. The folate polyglutamates in the diet are converted to monoglutamates by the action of the enzyme folate conjugase and the monoglutamates are converted to 5-methyltetrahydrofolate monoglutamate by the intestinal epithelial cell before entering the portal blood stream.

Storage and rate of loss of folates

The hepatic store of folate is normally greater than that of B_{12}, being about 8–20 mg. Folate is lost from the body in cells shed from the skin and intestinal epithelium, and in bile, urine, sweat and saliva. Folate is also lost by intracellular catabolism. The rate of loss of folate is approximately 1–2% of the total hepatic stores per day, a rate which is 10–20 times greater than the rate of loss of B_{12}. Since the minimum amount of folate required to be absorbed per day is about 100 times

Table 5.4 Causes of folate deficiency.

Inadequate dietary intake
Malabsorption
Coeliac disease, jejunal resection, tropical sprue
Increased requirement
Pregnancy, premature infants, chronic haemolytic anaemias, myelofibrosis, various malignant diseases
Increased loss
Long-term dialysis, congestive heart failure, acute liver disease
Complex mechanism
Anticonvulsant therapy,* ethanol abuse*

Note: * Only some cases with macrocytosis are folate deficient.

greater than that of B_{12}, and because folate turns over more rapidly than B_{12}, signs of folate deficiency appear much more rapidly than those of B_{12} deficiency. Thus, mildly megaloblastic haemopoiesis developed 5 months after a normal person was put on a folate-deficient diet, whereas it is known that after total gastrectomy, anaemia due to B_{12} deficiency does not develop for 2 years or more.

Factors causing folate deficiency

These are summarized in Table 5.4.

Inadequate diet

Megaloblastic anaemia due to inadequate intake of folate may be seen in the poor, some elderly people, the mentally disturbed, chronic alcoholics and infants fed on goat's milk which is low in folate (goat's milk anaemia).

Malabsorption

Since folate is absorbed in the upper part of the small intestine, diseases that affect this part, such as coeliac disease and tropical sprue, may cause megaloblastic anaemia due to folate deficiency. Jejunal resection may also be followed by folate deficiency. In these malabsorption syndromes, folate deficiency is commonly associated with iron deficiency. This is because iron is absorbed by the same region of the small bowel as folate.

Increased requirement

Folate deficiency and megaloblastic anaemia are found whenever there is an increased demand for folate that is not met by absorption from an adequate diet. The increased requirement for folate may result from increased nucleic acid synthesis (e.g. pregnancy and chronic haemolytic anaemia) or from increased loss of folate from the body (e.g. infection with sustained pyrexia or desquamating skin diseases such as psoriasis).

Megaloblastic anaemia of pregnancy

Before the use of folate supplements during pregnancy, macrocytic anaemia due to folate deficiency was found in 0.5–5% of all pregnancies in the UK. However, examination of the bone marrow during pregnancy revealed that megaloblastic haemopoiesis was even more common, being found in about one-third of cases. The diagnosis of megaloblastic anaemia is usually made after the 36th week of gestation or during the first 4 weeks of the postpartum period. The prevalence of megaloblastic anaemia of pregnancy is much higher in some developing countries than in the UK.

The chief cause of folate deficiency in pregnancy is the greatly increased DNA and RNA synthesis associated with the growth of the fetus, placenta and uterus, and the expansion of the red cell mass of the mother. It has been calculated that folate requirements increase approximately 3 times during pregnancy. Several subsidiary factors also play a part. About one-third of patients have anorexia and consequently a reduced food intake. There also appears to be a reduction in folate absorption during pregnancy, and an increase in folate requirement may result from urinary infection.

Diagnosis of folate deficiency

The haematological features of folate deficiency are macrocytosis with or without anaemia, hypersegmentation of circulating neutrophil granulocytes and megaloblastic haemopoiesis (p. 63). In order to establish that these changes are caused by folate deficiency rather than by any of the other causes of megaloblastic haemopoiesis, it is necessary to establish that the patient has reduced folate stores. This is usually done by measuring red cell folate levels. Serum folate levels are less reliable than red cell folate levels in assessing folate stores as they are readily affected by a short period of negative folate balance. However, even a low red cell folate level cannot on its own be considered proof of folate deficiency since low values are found in 60% of B_{12}-deficient patients. In practice therefore the diagnosis of folate deficiency requires not only the finding of a low red cell folate level in the appropriate clinical setting, but also the exclusion of B_{12} deficiency by demonstrating a normal serum B_{12} level, or in those patients with borderline or low serum vitamin B_{12} levels, a normal result with the Schilling test. Folate-deficient patients have raised serum levels of homocysteine but not of methylmalonic acid, whilst B_{12}-deficient patients have raised levels of both metabolites. However, such measurements are only made in a few specialist laboratories.

A simple but infrequently used method of establishing the diagnosis of folate deficiency is to demonstrate a haematological response to daily injections of physiological doses of folic acid (e.g. 200 μg daily); no response occurs in B_{12} deficiency. It is noteworthy that pharmacological doses of folic acid (5 mg daily by mouth) cause a temporary correction of the anaemia in B_{12} deficiency. However, if folate therapy is continued for more than 3 months, the anaemia recurs and neurological damage may be precipitated.

The cause of the folate deficiency is determined by taking a detailed dietary history and by performing tests of small intestinal function (including duodenal biopsy) when appropriate.

Treatment of folate deficiency

In an adult, macrocytosis or megaloblastic anaemia due to folate deficiency should be treated with 5 mg folic acid daily by mouth. The duration of treatment depends on the underlying disease but should, in any case, be at least 3 months. The initial haematological response is a reticulocytosis which peaks on the fifth to seventh day. The Hb concentration must be followed until it reaches the normal range, because a few patients, especially those with the malabsorption syndrome, may also be B_{12} or iron deficient; this can be detected by an incomplete rise in the Hb level. Such patients show a second response when vitamin B_{12} or iron is added to their treatment.

Folate and neural tube defects

There is an important relationship between folate and neural tube defects (e.g. spina bifida, anencephaly) that is not fully understood. In women who have had an infant with a neural tube defect, the incidence of such a defect in a subsequent pregnancy is reduced by about 70% by the administration of 4 mg folic acid daily given orally before conception and during the first 12 weeks of pregnancy. The dosage recommended to prevent the first occurrence of a neural tube defect is lower, being 400 μg per day.

Folate, vascular disease and cancer

Elevated homocysteine levels found in folate deficiency are a risk factor for coronary artery disease, cerebrovascular episodes and arterial peripheral vascular disease. There is also limited epidemiological evidence linking folate deficiency with an increased prevalence of dysplasias and colon cancer.

Disturbances in vitamin B_{12} or folate metabolism

N_2O disturbs B_{12} metabolism by oxidizing and inactivating methylcobalamin. Continuous exposure of patients to a mixture of 50% N_2O and 50% O_2 for 5–24 h often induces mild megaloblastic changes in the marrow. Intermittent exposure to N_2O for prolonged periods has caused a neuropathy in dentists working with, or addicted to, this gas. Drugs which inhibit dihydrofolate reductase (e.g. methotrexate and pyrimethamine) cause macrocytosis and megaloblastic changes by interfering with the regeneration of 5,10-methylenetetrahydrofolate from dihydrofolate. Megaloblastic haemopoiesis is also seen in some rare congenital disorders of vitamin B_{12} and

Table 5.5 Vitamin B_{12}-independent and folate-independent causes of macrocytosis with megaloblastic haemopoiesis.

Abnormalities of nucleic acid synthesis
Drug therapy
Antipurines (mercaptopurine, azathioprine)
Antipyrimidines (fluorouracil, zydovudine (AZT))
Others (hydroxyurea)
Orotic aciduria
Uncertain aetiology
Myelodysplastic syndromes,* erythroleukaemia
Some congenital dyserythropoietic anaemias

Note: * Some patients show normoblastic erythropoiesis.

Table 5.6 Causes of vitamin B_{12}- and folate-independent macrocytosis with normoblastic erythropoiesis.

Normal neonates (physiological)
Chronic alcoholism*
Myelodysplastic syndromes*
Chronic liver disease*
Hypothyroidism
Normal pregnancy
Therapy with anticonvulsant drugs*
Haemolytic anaemia
Chronic lung disease (with hypoxia)
Hypoplastic and aplastic anaemia
Myeloma

Note: * Some patients show B_{12}- and folate-independent megaloblastic erythropoiesis.

folate metabolism or of the B_{12} transport protein in plasma, transcobalamin II.

Vitamin B_{12}- and folate-independent causes of megaloblastic haemopoiesis

A list of conditions causing megaloblastic haemopoiesis by mechanisms unrelated to B_{12} or folate is given in Table 5.5. The drugs listed interfere with nucleic acid synthesis. Orotic aciduria is a rare inherited disorder in which megaloblastic anaemia develops because of a reduced activity of enzymes involved in the conversion of orotic acid to uridine monophosphate. This leads to an impairment in the supply of pyrimidine bases for incorporation into DNA and RNA.

Macrocytosis associated with normoblastic erythropoiesis

The conditions in which high MCVs may be associated with normoblastic erythropoiesis are listed in Table 5.6. The most common of these, and indeed the commonest cause of macrocytosis in the UK, is chronic alcohol abuse.

Chronic alcoholism

Many individuals with macrocytosis that is not due to B_{12} or folate deficiency consume excess quantities of alcohol. The level of alcohol consumption that induces macrocytosis varies considerably in different individuals. Only about 35%

of individuals who consume 100–800 g (mean 380 g) alcohol per day (i.e. an average of a bottle of spirits or its equivalent each day) develop MCVs above the normal range. Although some chronic alcoholics suffer from folate deficiency due to inadequate intake, the majority have neither B_{12} or folate deficiency, nor anaemia. When folate stores are adequate, erythropoiesis is usually normoblastic, not megaloblastic. It has been suggested that the macrocytosis is due to a toxic effect of acetaldehyde on erythroblasts. The acetaldehyde is probably generated locally by oxidation of ethanol by bone marrow macrophages. MCV values return to normal 2–3 months after stopping the high alcohol intake.

Haemolytic anaemia

Some patients with haemolytic anaemia develop increasing macrocytosis and megaloblastic haemopoiesis due to folate deficiency (p. 74). Other patients develop macrocytosis by a mechanism that is unrelated to folate deficiency. In the latter, the macrocytosis is associated with normoblastic erythropoiesis and is a manifestation of greatly accelerated erythropoiesis. The reticulocytes produced under these circumstances are larger than normal and mature into macrocytes that differ from those seen in B_{12} or folate deficiency in having rounded rather than oval outlines.

Hypothyroidism

There is a high frequency of thyroid and parietal cell antibodies in both hypothyroidism and pernicious anaemia and about 10% of all patients with hypothyroidism have pernicious anaemia. Patients with hypothyroidism may also develop macrocytosis by a mechanism that is based not on B_{12} or folate deficiency but on the deficiency of thyroxine. About one-quarter of patients with hypothyroidism (without associated pernicious anaemia) have an MCV above the normal range. Following the administration of thyroxine, all patients, including those whose MCV is within the normal range, show a fall in MCV.

Anticonvulsant drugs

A high MCV is seen in some patients receiving phenytoin sodium (with or without other anticonvulsant drugs) and this may be associated either with megaloblastic or normoblastic erythropoiesis. In a proportion of patients with megaloblastic changes, the macrocytosis is caused by folate deficiency and such patients are often anaemic. In the other patients with megaloblastic changes, and in all patients with normoblastic erythropoiesis, the macrocytosis is caused by an unknown mechanism independent of B_{12} and folate abnormalities; such patients are usually not anaemic.

Chapter 6

Conditions Associated with White Cell Abnormalities

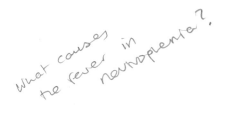

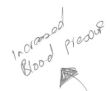

Learning objectives

- To understand the meaning of the terms leucopenia, neutropenia, leucocytosis, lymphopenia and lymphocytosis.
- To understand the significance of neutropenic sepsis and the importance of early identification and treatment.
- To know the common disorders associated with atypical lymphocytes in the blood particularly Epstein–Barr virus (EBV) infection.

Leucopenia

The terms 'leucopenia' and 'neutropenia' are used to describe a reduction in the total white cell count and neutrophil count, respectively, to values below their normal ranges. The term 'lymphopenia' are used when the lymphocyte count is subnormal.

Neutropenia

Neutrophils are highly motile cells which are required to maintain the integrity of mucosal surfaces and prevent overwhelming bacterial infection (see Chapter 1). There is a substantial risk of serious infection when the neutrophil count

Lecture Notes: Haematology, by NC Hughes-Jones, SN Wickramsinghe, CSR Hatton © 2008 Blackwell Publishing, ISBN: 9781405180504

falls below 0.5×10^9/L. The first symptom of neutropenia is sore throat (mucositis) and fever. Breakdown of the gastrointestinal mucosa may lead to Gram-negative septicaemia, hypotension and death (*neutropenic sepsis*). The management of neutropenic sepsis requires rapid assessment; urgent investigations including blood cultures and immediate use of intravenous antibiotics and adequate hydration. If the fever persists a programme of planned progressive therapy is used (Fig. 6.1). Patients with prolonged neutropenia are particularly prone to develop fungal infections, notably *Candida* and *Aspergillus*. *Candida* species usually affect the mouth and other mucosal surfaces, whereas *Aspergillus* species tend to cause invasive pulmonary disease.

Selective neutropenia (neutropenia without other cytopenias) may occur in a large number of conditions (Table 6.1). Cytotoxic drugs and radiotherapy cause a predictable neutropenia. Some combination chemotherapy regimens can lead to predictable neutropenia lasting days to weeks. Patients undergoing such treatment who become febrile require support with broad spectrum intravenous antibiotics and antifungal agents based on (planned progressive therapy) outlined above. Other drugs (Table 6.1), for example carbimazole, used to treat hyperthyroidism, and some antimalarial drugs are associated with idiosyncratic neutropenia. Patients taking these drugs should be warned about the remote

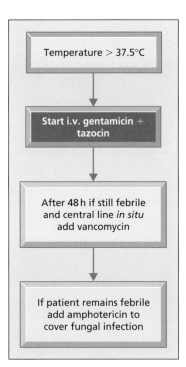

Figure 6.1 Planned progressive therapy for febrile patients with neutropaena (<0.5 × 10^9 L).

Table 6.1 The causes of selective neutropenia.

Physiological
Neutropenia in blacks (see p. 6).

Certain drugs
Anti-inflammatory drugs: indomethacin, oxyphenbutazone, phenylbutazone, sodium aurothiomalate.
Antibacterial drugs: chloramphenicol, co-trimoxazole (sulphamethoxazole–trimethoprim), other sulphonamides.
Some anticonvulsants, oral hypoglycaemic agents, antithyroid drugs, antimalarial drugs, tranquillizers, antidepressants and antihistamines.

Infections
Bacterial: overwhelming pyogenic infections, brucellosis, typhoid, miliary tuberculosis.
Some viral, protozoal and fungal infections.

Immune neutropenia
Systemic lupus erythematosus (SLE), Felty's syndrome, autoimmune neutropenia, neonatal alloimmune neutropenia, aminopyrine-induced agranulocytosis.

Miscellaneous
Hypothyroidism, hypopituitarism, cyclical neutropenia, familial benign chronic neutropenia.

but possible risk of neutropenia and advised to stop the drug should they develop a sore throat or fever.

Leucocytosis

An increase in the total white cell count is described as a leucocytosis. The term 'neutrophil leucocytosis' is used to describe an absolute increase in the total number of neutrophils in the peripheral blood (also known as neutrophilia). Eosinophilia is the term used to describe an absolute increase in the number of eosinophils. Similarly, basophilia is the term used to describe an absolute increase in the basophil count. Monocytosis describes an increase in the absolute monocyte count.

Neutrophil leucocytosis

The causes of neutrophil leucocytosis are shown in Table 6.2. Bacterial infection is an important cause but many varied insults will elevate the

Table 6.2 The causes of neutrophil leucocytosis.

Physiological
Neonates, exercise, pregnancy, parturition, lactation.

Pathological
Acute infections: especially by pyogenic bacteria.
Acute inflammation not caused by infections: surgery, burns, infarcts, crush injuries, rheumatoid arthritis, myositis, vasculitis.
Acute haemorrhage and acute haemolysis.
Metabolic: uraemia, diabetic ketoacidosis, gout, acute thyrotoxicosis.
Non-haematological malignancies: carcinoma, melanoma.
Lymphoma
Chronic myeloproliferative disorders: chronic myeloid leukaemia, polycythaemia vera, myelofibrosis.
Drugs: adrenaline, corticosteroids, G-CSF and GM-CSF.
Miscellaneous: convulsions, paroxysmal tachycardia, electric shock, postneutropenic rebound neutrophilia, postsplenectomy.

Temperature > 37.5°C

Start i.v. gentamicin + tazocin

After 48 h if still febrile and central line in situ add vancomycin

If patient remains febrile add amphotericin to cover fungal infection

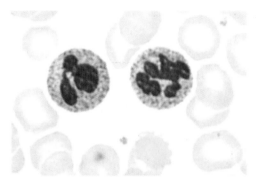

Figure 6.2 Toxic granulation in two neutrophils from a patient with an infection.

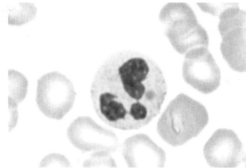

Figure 6.3 Round, pale-blue Döhle body near the nucleus of a neutrophil from a patient with extensive burns. Döhle bodies may also be oval or rod shaped and are more frequently seen at the periphery than at the centre of the cell.

neutrophil count. In addition, metamyelocytes and small numbers of myelocytes may be present in severe infection — 'shift to the left.' Neutrophils may show toxic granulation (Fig. 6.2), or Döhle bodies (Fig. 6.3), or both. Toxic granules are abnormally coarse, reddish violet (azurophilic) granules, which are diffusely distributed throughout the cytoplasm. Döhle bodies are 1–2μm long, pale greyish blue cytoplasmic inclusions (Romanowsky stain). A 'shift to the left,' toxic granulation and Döhle bodies reflect accelerated neutrophil production and may be seen not only in acute infection but also in non-infective inflammatory states (e.g. severe burns), in normal pregnancy and in patients with various malignant neoplasms.

The neutrophil leucocytosis seen with steroid administration and after exercise is caused by a rapid shift of neutrophils from the marginated to the circulating granulocyte pool (p. 6).

Abnormalities of granulocyte morphology and function

There are a number of inherited conditions causing abnormalities in granulocyte morphology or function or both. The essential features of some of these are summarized in Table 6.3. The most common acquired abnormalities of neutrophil morphology include 'shift to the left,' hypersegmentation of the nucleus (p. 63), toxic granulation, Döhle bodies, hypogranularity and the acquired Pelger–Huët anomaly (p. 127).

Eosinophilia

Eosinophilia is usually caused by allergic disorders or parasitic infestation. Asthma, eczema and drugs are the commonest causes but there are many others, some of which are listed in Table 6.4.

Basophilia

Basophilia is an uncommon finding and should raise the possibility of a myeloid haematological malignancy such as chronic myeloid leukaemia or myelodysplasia. Other causes include myxoedema and hypersensitivity reactions.

Monocytosis

A high monocyte count is seen in many inflammatory disorders and malignant states. A high monocyte count is also found in chronic myelomonocytic leukaemia, one of the myelodysplastic disorders (p. 127).

Lymphocytosis and lymphopenia

An increase in the blood lymphocyte count is called a *lymphocytosis*. This is defined as a lymphocyte count greater than 4.0×10^9/L. *Lymphopenia* refers to a decrease in the number of circulating lymphocytes and is defined as a total lymphocyte count below 1×10^9/L. In normal blood most lymphocytes are CD4+ T cells. Important causes

Table 6.3 Some inherited abnormalities of neutrophil morphology or function or both.

Condition	Inheritance, prevalence	Characteristics
Pelger–Huët anomaly	Autosomal dominant 1:1000–10,000	Heterozygotes have bilobed spectacle-like neutrophil nuclei, homozygotes have round or oval neutrophil nuclei; asymptomatic
Neutrophil myeloperoxidase deficiency	Autosomal recessive 1:2000	Detected during automated differential counting based on cytochemistry; usually asymptomatic
Chediak–Higashi syndrome	Autosomal recessive	Giant granules in leucocytes, neutropenia, thrombocytopaenia, partial albinism, hepatosplenomegaly, death in infancy or early childhood from infection and haemorrhage
Chronic granulomatous disease	Majority X-linked, some autosomal recessive	Normal neutrophil morphology, inability to kill ingested microorganisms due to absence of cytochrome b_{558} or other components of the respiratory chain (p. 7) leading to impaired superoxide generation, recurrent granulomatous lesions from early childhood

Table 6.4 The causes of eosinophilia.

Parasitic infestations: Filariasis, hookworm, ascariasis, strongyloidiasis, schistosomiasis, toxocariasis, trichinosis, hydatid cyst, scabies.
Allergic disorders: Bronchial asthma, hay fever, allergic vasculitis, Stevens–Johnson syndrome, drug sensitivity (e.g. chlorpromazine, penicillin, sulphonamides).
Recovery from acute infection
Skin diseases: Eczema, psoriasis, pemphigus, dermatitis herpetiformis.
Pulmonary eosinophilia: Loeffler's syndrome (pulmonary infiltration with eosinophilia).
Polyarteritis nodosa
Chronic myeloid leukaemia, eosinophilic leukaemia (rare).
Other malignant diseases: Hodgkin lymphoma, angioimmunoblastic lymphoma, carcinoma (usually with metastases).
Idiopathic hypereosinophilic syndrome.

of lymphocytopaenia include acquired immune deficiency syndrome (AIDS), radiotherapy, chemotherapy and steroid therapy. A transient low lymphocyte count is often found in patients with severe infection.

Transient lymphocytosis

The morphological features of lymphocytes enable the distinction between reactive and malignant causes. The most common cause of reactive lymphocytosis is infectious mononucleosis (see below). Lymphocytosis may be associated with other viral infections such as cytomegalovirus (CMV), hepatitis and human immunodeficiency virus (HIV) (early stages). Whooping cough (*Bordetella pertussis*) is an important cause of lymphocytosis in children.

Persistent lymphocytosis

Persistent lymphocytosis is suggestive of an underlying lymphoproliferative disorder and requires further characterization. There are benign causes but in older persons the most common cause is B-cell chronic lymphocytic leukaemia. The profile of antigens expressed by cells can be determined by the technique of *flow cytometry*. The antigen profile of lymphocytes allows differentiation between malignant and benign conditions and also allows characterization of individual cells into B- and T-cell subtypes.

Flow cytometry: a technique for identification of cells in suspension

Flow cytometry is a technique used to characterize cells, usually in the peripheral blood or in bone marrow aspirate samples. It is a method which allows the detection of specific antigens on

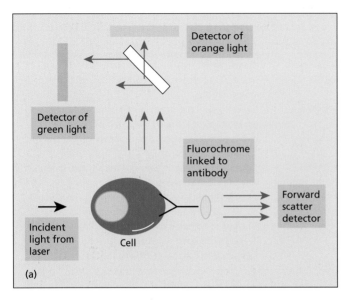

(a)

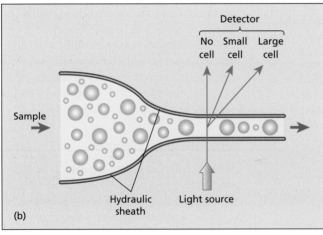

(b)

Figure 6.4 (a) Schematic diagram to illustrate general principles of flow cytometry. (b) Schematic diagram showing how cells are presented to a laser light beam by hydrodynamic focusing.

the cell surface or, if the cell is made permeable, in its cytoplasm and nucleus. This is achieved by measuring fluorescence and light scatter of cells as they flow in a coaxial stream through a beam of intense light. The fluorescence generated may be 'self-generated' autofluorescence, due to cytochromes and other intracellular components, or may arise because the cells have been prelabelled with fluorochromes conjugated to antigen-binding antibodies. It is this latter technique which permits the detection of specific cell surface antigens. Most flow cytometers use an argon laser to excite

fluorochromes such as fluorescein isothiocyanate (FITC, green), phycoerythrin (PE, orange) and peridinin chlorophyll protein (PerCP, red), which are bound to cell surface antigens. The different emission spectra of the fluorochromes allow cells labelled with FITC to be distinguished from cells labelled with PE or PerCP (Fig. 6.4), and this in turn enables cells carrying specific antigens to be defined.

The deflection of the laser beam by the cell also gives information about the size and granularity of the cell. Forward scatter of light relates to the size of a cell, whereas side scatter (SSC) relates to

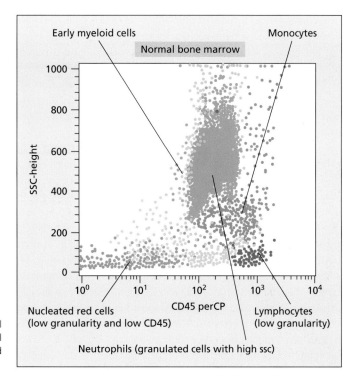

Figure 6.5 Flow cytometry of normal bone marrow after incubating normal bone marrow cells with PerCP-labelled anti-CD45 antibody.

the granularity of the cell. Figure 6.5 shows flow cytometry performed on a normal bone marrow incubated with anti-CD45 antibody labelled with the fluorochromes PerCP (CD45 is an antigen present on most haemopoietic cells apart from nucleated red cells, some blasts cells and plasma cells). It demonstrates the ability to separate different populations of cells within the bone marrow sample.

Infectious mononucleosis

This is a syndrome characterized by the appearance of reactive lymphocytes in the peripheral blood caused by infection (Fig. 6.6). The commonest causative agent is the EBV. Other agents include *Toxoplasma gondii*, CMV and HIV.

EBV infection

EBV infection is caused by close mucosal contact (e.g. kissing an carrier). The virus infects the respiratory epithelium causing pharyngitis, often with a significant exudate on the tonsillar bed. The virus enters the blood leading to lymphadenopathy,

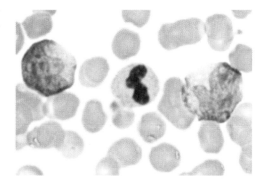

Figure 6.6 Two atypical mononuclear cells (reactive lymphocytes) and a neutrophil from a patient with glandular fever. Although the atypical mononuclear cells are similar in size to the monocyte in Fig. 1.4(c), their cytoplasm is much more basophilic and not vacuolated.

fever and hepatosplenomegaly. Liver function tests may be abnormal. The illness is usually self-limiting but can lead to persistent lassitude and fatigue. Patients given amoxycillin may develop a florid rash that is almost diagnostic in this clinical setting.

A characteristic feature of this illness is the development of antibodies capable of agglutinating red cells of other species — horse red cells or sheep red cells. Non-specific antibodies can be absorbed out using guinea-pig kidney cells allowing the specific antibodies to be titrated against sheep red cells; this is the basis of the Paul–Bunnell test. The monospot test uses a similar agglutination reaction for the detection of heterophile antibodies against horse red blood cells. When positive the monospot test is highly suggestive of infectious mononucleosis caused by EBV. It is also well known that some patients develop autoimmune complications such as autoimmune haemolytic anaemia and immune thrombocytopaenia.

The EBV virus, having been shed from the pharyngeal mucosa, infects B-lymphocytes causing them to proliferate. This is followed by activation of T cells, mainly CD8+ cytotoxic T cells, which control the B-cell proliferation. The 'reactive' or atypical lymphocytes characteristic of this condition consist mainly of these T cells. Infected B cells harbouring EBV persist throughout life. Asymptomatic carriers periodically shed virus from the pharynx thereby ensuring that the virus is passed on to non-immune persons. Patients who receive immunosuppressive therapy following renal, heart/lung or bone marrow transplantation may lose the T-cell control necessary to control the EBV-infected B cells. The resulting B-cell lymphoproliferation may involve lymph nodes or extranodal sites resulting in a condition known as a post-transplant lymphoproliferative disorder or PTLD.

Infection and immunity

Virus infection

EBV is transmitted via saliva and establishes replicative infection within cells of the oropharynx where it expresses lytic cycle proteins. It goes on to establish latent infection within B cells (Fig. 6.7). During the primary phase of infection all the EBV latent proteins are expressed within B cells (latency III programme of gene transcription). Following primary infection the numbers of infected B cells fall and expression of the viral

latent proteins is downregulated (latency I programme of gene transcription). In this form the virus can evade the host's immune response and the infection is therefore persistent. Periodic reactivation of EBV may occur resulting in low level virus replication in the oropharynx, virus shedding in saliva and transmission to other hosts.

Immune response

Primary infection stimulates a vigorous immune response with the expansion of CD8+ T cells specific for the EBV lytic cycle and latent proteins, and a smaller expansion of CD4+ T cells. As primary infection is controlled, the number of EBV-specific T cells falls; although a significant proportion of the T-cell pool remains committed to recognition of EBV. During primary infection the humoral response includes IgM antibodies specific for the viral capsid antigens (VCA) and IgG antibodies specific for the nuclear antigen, EBNA2. Neutralizing IgG antibodies, specific for a membrane antigen (MA), gp350, and IgG antibodies specific for a different nuclear antigen, EBNA1, arise later in the course of infection.

CMV infection

CMV infection usually causes a milder pharyngitis but with a higher fever and greater splenomegaly than is found in EBV mononucleosis. The importance of CMV is in immunocompromised persons, most notably in the post-transplant setting where an absence of controlling T cells can lead to life-threatening complications such as CMV pneumonitis.

Toxoplasmosis

Toxoplasmosis often produces prominent lymphadenopathy. Fever in this condition may be absent. The finding of IgM toxoplasma antibodies is diagnostic.

HIV

HIV can present with very many different haematological manifestations, but amongst these is a 'mononucleosis-like' syndrome. Autoimmune

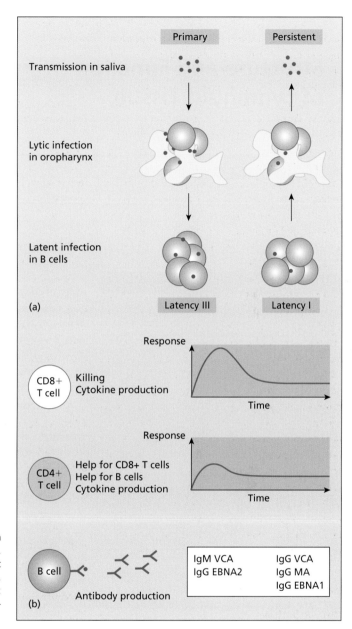

Figure 6.7 Features of EBV infection and the resulting immune response. IgM antibody to VCA is diagnostic of a recent or continuing infection. *Notes*: VCA — viral capsid antigens; EBNA — Epstein–Barr nuclear antigens; MA — membrane antigen.

haemolytic anaemia, immune thrombocytopaenia and thrombotic thrombocytopaenic purpura may also occur in patients with HIV.

Leukoerythroblastic reaction

The characteristic feature is the presence of nucleated red cells as well as immature white cells (mainly myelocytes) in the peripheral blood film. The finding is important as it may be seen when the bone marrow is infiltrated with malignant cells, either haematological or non-haematological. A bone marrow aspirate and trephine biopsy may establish the diagnosis. Other causes include hypoxia and sepsis.

Chapter 7

Structure and Function of Lymphoid Tissue

Learning objectives

- To understand the components of the immune system.
- To have a basic understanding of the structure of lymph nodes.
- To know that it is immunoglobulin gene rearrangement that defines a B cell.
- To know that it is T-cell receptor (TCR) gene rearrangement that defines a T cell.
- To understand that malignant disorders derive from the recognizable normal components.

Lymphocytes can be divided into three main classes of effector cell: B-lymphocytes, T-lymphocytes and natural killer (NK) cells, all of which derive from precursor cells in the bone marrow (Fig. 7.1).

B cells are the effector cells of *humoral immunity (antibody production)* and are thought to arise in the bone marrow where they begin life as a blast cell and mature in peripheral lymphoid tissue (e.g. lymph nodes, gut and bone marrow), to become antibody-producing *plasma cells*. This maturation involves rearrangement and mutation of their immunoglobulin genes allowing expression of

Lecture Notes: Haematology, by NC Hughes-Jones, SN Wickramsinghe, CSR Hatton © 2008 Blackwell Publishing, ISBN: 9781405180504

surface and secreted immunoglobulin with a wide range of antigen-binding specificities.

T cells are the effector cells of *cell-mediated immunity*. Precursors of T cells migrate to the thymus where they develop into CD4 (helper) and CD8 (suppressor/cytotoxic) cells, before migrating to other lymphoid organs, including the spleen and bone marrow.

NK cells mediate *natural killer cell function*. These cells lack B- or T-cell markers and were previously referred to as null cells. They have a characteristic morphology, being generally larger than other lymphocytes and having small granules in their cytoplasm ('large granular lymphocytes') (Fig. 1.6).

Lymph node structure

Lymph nodes contain densely packed T- and B-lymphocytes, organized in a manner which allows the presentation of antigen to produce an effective immune response. In addition to having a blood supply, lymph nodes receive 'afferent' lymphatic vessels which drain antigen-rich lymph from the tissues. Within the unstimulated lymph node, resting B cells are organized into structures called *primary follicles* (Fig. 7.2). When exposed to antigen (e.g. from microorganisms) these structures enlarge and *germinal centres* develop, comprising proliferating B cells lying within a meshwork of 'follicular dentritic cells.' Surrounding the

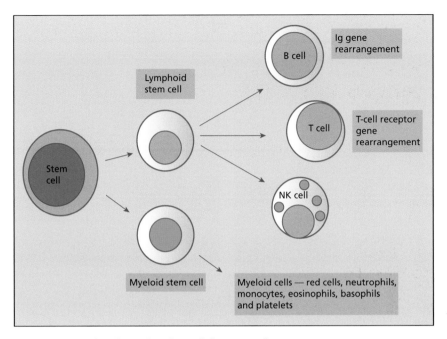

Figure 7.1 The derivation of B cells, T cells and NK cells from stem cells.

follicles there are sheets of lymphocytes which become increasingly rich in T cells toward the lymph node medulla. The medulla contains different types of lymphocytes, including plasma cells.

Other lymphoid tissue

Lymphoid tissue is found in many sites other than lymph nodes. These sites include tissues directly exposed to external pathogens (e.g. the respiratory and gastrointestinal tracts) and also 'central sites' such as the bone marrow and spleen. Plasma cells are found in many lymphoid tissues, particularly at sites where they can secrete immunoglobulin into the circulation or mucous secretions (e.g. into the respiratory or gastrointestinal tracts).

Immunoglobulin structure and gene rearrangement

The defining feature of B-cell development is the production of immunoglobulin with a wide range of antibody specificities. Immunoglobulins are made up of two identical heavy chains and two identical light chains (either κ or λ) (Fig. 7.3). The five major classes of immunoglobulin — IgA, IgG, IgM, IgD and IgE — are defined by their heavy chains (α, γ, μ, δ and ε). The two heavy chains and two light chains are held together in a Y-shaped structure. The amino terminal portions of the heavy and light chains are known as 'variable' regions (V_H or V_L) since differences in their amino acid sequence create unique antigen-binding sites, each of which can recognize a different epitope. In contrast, the carboxy terminal regions are the 'constant' regions (C_H or C_L) because their structure is similar for all immunoglobulins of the same class. The enzyme papain cleaves the immunoglobulin molecule into an Fc fragment consisting of the carboxy terminal regions of the heavy chain and two Fab fragments containing the antigen-binding site. A number of cell types possess Fc receptors that can bind the Fc portion of immunoglobulin molecules.

Human plasma contains all types of immunoglobulin, but IgG is present at the highest concentration. IgA is the second commonest type

87

Primary follicle

Secondary follicle

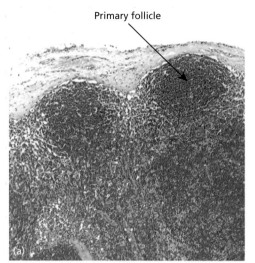
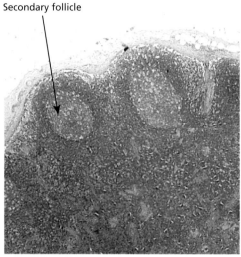

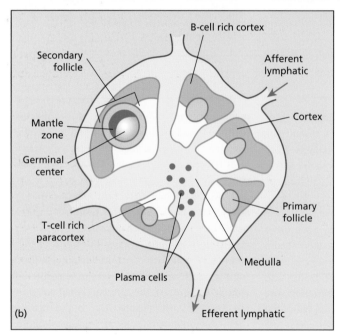

B-cell rich cortex

Secondary
follicle

Afferent
lymphatic

Mantle
zone

Cortex

Germinal
center

T-cell rich
paracortex

Primary
follicle

Medulla

Plasma cells

Efferent lymphatic

Figure 7.2 (a) Histological section through a lymph node and (b) drawing of a stylized lymph node.

of immunoglobulin and is found at mucosal surfaces in the gut and the respiratory system. IgM represents only 6% of the immunoglobulin found in plasma and is the antibody most commonly produced during a primary immune response. IgM has a very large molecular weight (c. 900,000 kDa) and is pentameric in structure. The high molecular weight of IgM can be very relevant in disorders such as Waldenstrom's macroglobulinaemia where large amounts of secreted monoclonal protein can cause a considerable increase in blood viscosity.

Light chains

These are low molecular weight proteins (23 kDa) and are present in a κ:λ ratio of 2:1. The κ gene is situated on chromosome 2, while the λ gene is located on chromosome 22.

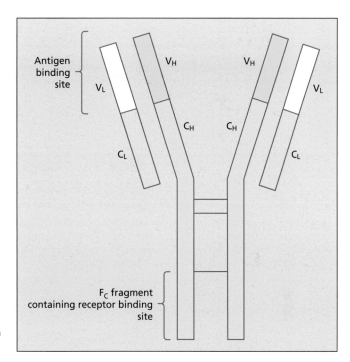

Figure 7.3 Schematic model of an IgG molecule.

Heavy chains

The immunoglobulin heavy chain gene complex is located on chromosome 14. It consists of 100–200 heavy chain variable genes (V_H), at least 24 diversity genes, 6 junctional minigenes and exons that encode the heavy chain constant regions characteristic of each class (Fig. 7.4).

Antibody diversity

Immunoglobulin gene rearrangement is the mechanism by which a single variable gene (V_H or V_L) in either a heavy or light chain gene complex is juxtaposed to genes encoding the constant region (C_H or C_L), generating differences from one immunoglobulin molecule to another in antigen-binding specificities (Fig. 7.4). Diversity is increased by the introduction of randomly generated sequences as well as by mutations within the variable regions. In consequence,

a B-cell clone can synthesize immunoglobulin molecules with unique antigen-binding sites. It may be added that at different stages of differentiation, a single B cell can synthesize heavy chains with different constant regions but with the same variable regions and thus antigen specificity. Thus a B cell can start by expressing IgM but following antigen binding can produce IgG, IgA or IgE.

B-cell selection and maturation

B cells arising from progenitor cells in the bone marrow make their way to the germinal centre of lymphoid tissue where they encounter antigen already bound to dentritic reticulum cells. If the surface immunoglobulin (SIg) on the B cells binds this antigen, the cross linking provides a survival signal. Otherwise the B cells undergo apoptosis, a process that ensures selection of 'useful' B cells, which become memory B cell and plasma cells.

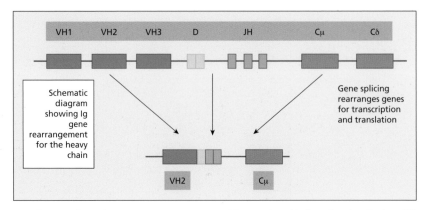

Figure 7.4 A diagram illustrating gene rearrangement enabling antigen-binding diversity. During differentiation, a single B cell can synthesize heavy chains with different constant regions coupled to the same variable region. The T-cell receptor (TCR) undergoes gene rearrangement in a very similar way in T cells. *Notes:* C — constant region gene, D — diversity genes, JH — joining sequences, V_H — variable genes.

T-lymphocyte antigen receptors

The antigen receptor on T cells (*T-cell receptor* or TCR) is formed from two polypeptide chains, usually α and β, and less commonly γ and δ. TCR molecules are very comparable in structure to immunoglobulin molecules and the diversity in their binding sites results from a similar process (e.g. the rearrangement of variable and constant region genes). Interaction of the TCR and a binding ligand results in T-cell activation and proliferation.

During differentiation, T cells migrate from the bone marrow to the thymus where they encounter major histocompatibility complex (MHC) class I molecules on the thymic epithelium. Any T cells that fail to recognize these molecules will die by apoptosis and the same fate awaits cells that bind with very high affinity. As a consequence the T cells that emerge from the thymus all carry TCRs with an intermediate affinity for 'self' MHC molecules. This ensures that they will subsequently continuously bind to (and disengage from) self-MHC molecules. However, if alteration of the MHC molecule by the presence of a peptide (e.g. from a virus) increases the affinity of TCR binding,

the cell presenting the peptide with the MHC molecule will become the target for specific recognition and killing.

Natural killer cells

NK cells differ from T cells in that they do not express TCRs but they are nevertheless capable of mediating cell lysis. This is achieved through surface receptors that suppress NK activity when they engage MHC molecules on a cell. However, the absence of MHC molecules on a cell removes this inhibition and the NK cells then initiate cytotoxic destruction of the target cell.

NK cells express FcγRIIIA (CD16) — a receptor that recognizes antibody on the surface of a cell — and thereby induce antibody-dependent cell-mediated cytotoxicity (ADCC). Furthermore, NK cell activation leads to the production of cytokines including interferon γ (IFN-γ), macrophage and granulocyte–macrophage colony-stimulating factor (M-CSF, GM-CSF), interleukin-3 (IL-3) and tumour necrosis factor α (TNF-α). These cytokines effect neutrophil recruitment and function, in addition to helping to activate the monocyte/macrophage system. NK cells can lyse virus-infected cells and may be able to lyse tumour cells.

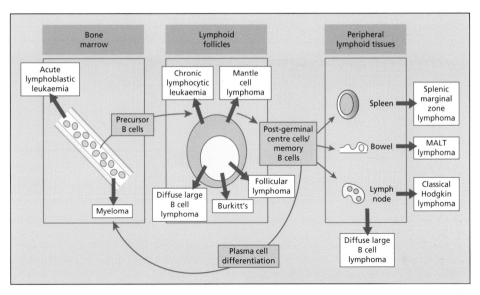

Figure 7.5 Lymphomas arise from 'normal cellular components' of the immune system. Pre-germinal centre cells may give rise to CLL or mantle cell lymphoma. The majority of other lymphomas arise from mutations in cells derived from the germinal centre or the post-germinal centre. *Source*: Courtesy of Professor David Mason.

Cellular origin of lymphomas

The vast majority of lymphomas are of B-cell origin; T-cell lymphoma only accounts for approximately 10% of all lymphomas. Lymphomas may arise from any of the stages of T-cell or B-cell maturation. Lymphoma cells have the distinctive morphology and immunophenotype of normal stages of differentiation, which allows them to be classified according to their postulated cell of origin. Figure 7.5 shows how the malignant B-cell disorders relate to the stages of maturation as B cells journey through the lymph nodes and other lymphoid structures.

Chapter 8

Lymphomas: General Principles

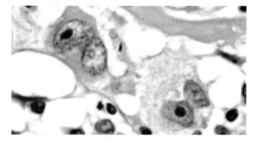

Figure 8.1 Two Reed–Sternberg cells — their presence defines Hodgkin lymphoma.

Lymphomas are *clonal malignant disorders* that derive from *lymphoid cells*, either precursor or mature T cells or B cells. They are divided into two broad categories, namely, *Hodgkin lymphoma* and *non-Hodgkin lymphoma*. Hodgkin lymphoma is diagnosed histologically by the presence of Reed–Sternberg cells (Fig. 8.1) within the appropriate cellular background (p. 103).

Lymphomas versus leukaemias

The distinction between lymphoma and leukaemia is somewhat artificial. Lymphomas are generally thought of as being 'solid' (lumps) whereas leukaemias are 'liquid' with malignant cells

spilling into the peripheral blood. Modern classifications are based on the cell of origin and define biological entities (e.g. follicular centre cells giving rise to follicular lymphoma, or cells from the mantle zone giving rise to mantle cell lymphoma). Note that in modern classifications lymphomas include some conditions that have malignant cells in the peripheral blood and are conventionally thought of as being a form of leukaemia. Thus, chronic lymphocytic leukaemia (CLL) and acute lymphoblastic leukaemia are now classified with the lymphomas.

Lymphomas

Aetiology and epidemiology

Lymphomas are more common in males and in older people. Marked variations in racial incidence,

Lecture Notes: Haematology, by NC Hughes-Jones, SN Wickramsinghe, CSR Hatton © 2008 Blackwell Publishing, ISBN: 9781405180504

histology and immunological subtypes occur around the world. The aetiology of lymphomas is generally unknown, though certain types are associated with specific infectious agents. Epstein–Barr virus (EBV) is present in over 90% of cases of endemic Burkitt's lymphoma. Human T-cell leukaemia virus 1 (HTLV-1), a retrovirus, is associated with a very aggressive form of T-cell lymphoma found in Japan and Caribbean countries, and some cases of gastric lymphoma are known to be triggered by infection with *Helicobacter pylori*.

Cytogenetics and molecular considerations

Cytogenetic analysis has identified a number of specific recurring abnormalities that are associated with certain lymphomas. The alteration of expression of genes involved in cell proliferation, cell differentiation and apoptosis result from these specific genetic alterations.

In 75% of Burkitt's lymphoma, translocation of the c-*MYC* gene on chromosome 8 close to the immunoglobulin heavy chain gene locus on chromosome 14, leads to upregulation and expression of the c-MYC protein, which causes cell proliferation and a failure of apoptosis (Fig. 8.2). This translocation t(8;14) is diagnostic of the condition. The remaining 25% of Burkitt's lymphomas involve translocations of c-*MYC* to the proximity of the genes coding the κ and λ light chains — t(2;8) and t(8;22). Identification of these genetic and molecular abnormalities not only sheds light on the mechanisms of disease, but provides valuable diagnostic information.

Such molecular subclassification allows the identification of lymphomas that have different clinical outcomes with treatment and therefore may help define treatment strategies. They may also identify specific molecular targets for treatment. *Gene expression profiling* (a technique capable of determining the expression of thousands of genes and allowing comparison of the gene expression of one malignant disorder to another using a *microarray*) is helping to identify subsets of lymphomas within the main categories. Diffuse large cell lymphoma is generally thought to be a heterogeneous collection of lymphomas and gene expression studies using microarrays have identified three distinctive patterns of gene expression. This work is at the research level but is likely to alter our perceptions about this and other malignant disorders. It may be that data on the expression of a relatively small number of genes from individual cases of lymphoma or leukaemia may be able to direct therapy.

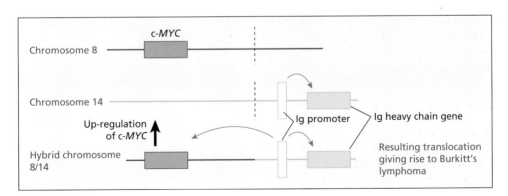

Figure 8.2 Upregulation of c-*MYC* in Burkitt's lymphoma. A translocation between chromosome 14 and chromosome 8 juxtaposes the c-*MYC* oncogene with the immunoglobulin heavy chain gene promoter, thereby up-regulating the oncogene c-*MYC* and driving the cell into cycle. The translocation of an oncogene to the vicinity of the Ig gene promoter is a common feature in B-cell lymphomas.

DNA microarray technology

DNA microarray technology allows the simultaneous analysis of the expression levels of thousands of genes in cells or tissues of interest.

The study of gene expression by DNA microarray technology is based on the hybridization of messenger RNA (mRNA) to a high-density array of immobilized target sequences, each corresponding to a specific gene. Sample mRNAs are labelled as a complex mixture, usually by incorporation of a fluorescent nucleotide. The labelled pool of sample mRNA is subsequently hybridized to the array, where each messenger will quantitatively hybridize to its complementary sequence. After washing, the fluorescence at each spot on the array is a quantitative measure corresponding to the expression level of the particular gene. The use of two differently labelled mRNA samples allows a quantitative comparison of gene expression in both samples (Fig. 8.3).

Microarrays can be used to compare gene expression in different cell types or tissue types, for example cancer versus normal cells, and to examine changes in gene expression at different stages in the cell cycle or during development. The examination of gene expression using microarray holds great promise for the identification of candidate genes involved in a variety of cell processes. The identification of new target genes and pathways should allow the development of specific molecular-based anticancer drugs. In addition, expression profiles will permit tumour classification into more homogenous groups and will help identify prognostic groups, as well as the identification of new clinically and biologically relevant tumour entities.

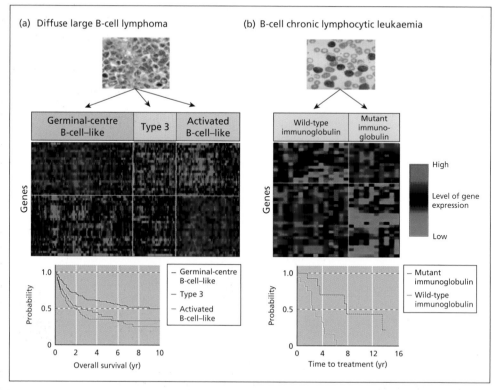

Figure 8.3 cDNA microarray containing 10,000 spots showing differential gene expression. *Notes*: Red — high gene expression; green — low gene expression.

High- and low-grade disease

Clinicians often divide lymphoid disorders into low and high grade (Table 8.1). High-grade lymphomas are those that are rapidly fatal if left untreated but can sometimes be cured with multiagent chemotherapy. Low-grade lymphomas generally have a low proliferation rate and can be controlled with mild chemotherapy but are incurable (Fig. 8.4).

Table 8.1 Examples of high- and low-grade lymphoid neoplasms.

Waldenstrom's macroglobulinaemia/immunocytoma	Low grade
Follicular lymphoma	Low grade
Chronic lymphocytic leukaemia	Low grade
Mantle cell lymphoma	Low grade
Diffuse large B-cell lymphoma	High grade
Acute lymphoblastic leukaemia/lymphoblastic lymphoma	High grade
Burkitt's lymphoma	High grade

The division of lymphomas into high or low grade is too imprecise to use as a definitive method for classifying lymphomas or directing treatment. Mantle cell lymphoma is an example of a low-grade lymphoma in terms of its low proliferation rate and incurability, but has the worst prognosis of any lymphoma. Low-grade lymphomas may transform into high-grade tumours that require treatment with combination chemotherapy (Fig. 8.5).

Clinical manifestations

Many lymphomas will present as a lump, in which case reaching the diagnosis is generally straightforward. However, some cases may present diagnostic difficulties. Lymphomas are great mimickers of other diseases. They present with weight loss, fever or sweats and are a serious consideration in a patient with pyrexia of unknown origin. Pruritus is another symptom that should alert the diagnosis of lymphoma. Lymphomas may cause obstruction of the bile duct (nodes in the porta hepatis), or block the renal outflow tract.

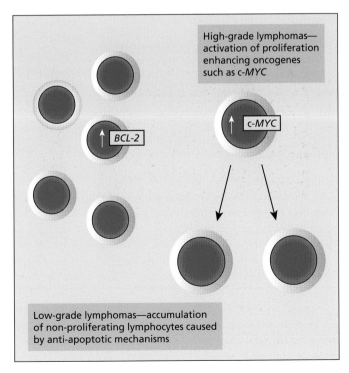

Figure 8.4 Schematic diagram to illustrate the molecular difference between 'low' and 'high' grade lymphomas.

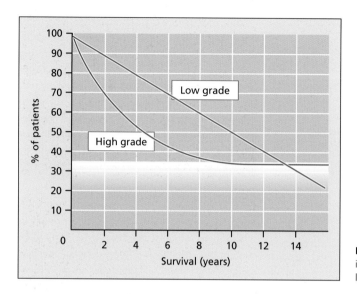

Figure 8.5 Schematic diagram showing outcome for low- and high-grade lymphoma.

Nodal and extranodal lymphomas

About 60% of lymphomas involve the lymph nodes; the remaining 40% may involve almost any organ of the body.

Diagnosis is made by biopsy

The diagnosis is based on the histological appearances of an enlarged lymph node or other affected tissue or the cytology of blood or cerebrospinal fluid (CSF), but this is usually backed up by immunophenotyping and other techniques (outlined below).

Immunophenotyping

The identification of cell-type-specific proteins using labelled antibodies may be very helpful for diagnosis. The process of categorizing the antigenic molecules and epitopes associated with human white cells began in the 1980s. Following a series of workshops, there is now an internationally agreed basis for the nomenclature of leucocyte molecules — the CD scheme.

For example, B cells express an array of different proteins not normally expressed by T cells and other haemopoietic cells. CD20 is one such molecule exclusively expressed on B cells during the middle stage of their development. The anti-CD20 antibody will bind to cells expressing CD20, thereby identifying the cell as being of B-cell origin. The function of CD20 is not fully known. CD19, CD22 and CD79 are other examples of B-cell-expressed molecules identified by antibody binding. The use of labelled antibodies against cells in suspension or on paraffin sections allows identification of expressed antigens (see also section 'Flow cytometry' in Chapter 6, p. 81) (Fig. 8.6).

Staging

Once the diagnosis of lymphoma has been made by biopsy or examination of blood, pleural fluid or perhaps CSF, staging should be undertaken (Table 8.2). *CT scanning* is the mainstay of staging (Fig. 8.7). Imaging will demonstrate the extent of enlarged lymph nodes, whether the liver and spleen are enlarged and whether other organs are involved. *Bone marrow biopsy* is important in non-Hodgkin lymphoma due to the high frequency of bone marrow involvement in this disorder. Hodgkin lymphoma rarely affects the bone marrow as its principal mode of spread is lymphatic rather than haematogenous. Measurement of serum lactate dehydrogenase (LDH) is important

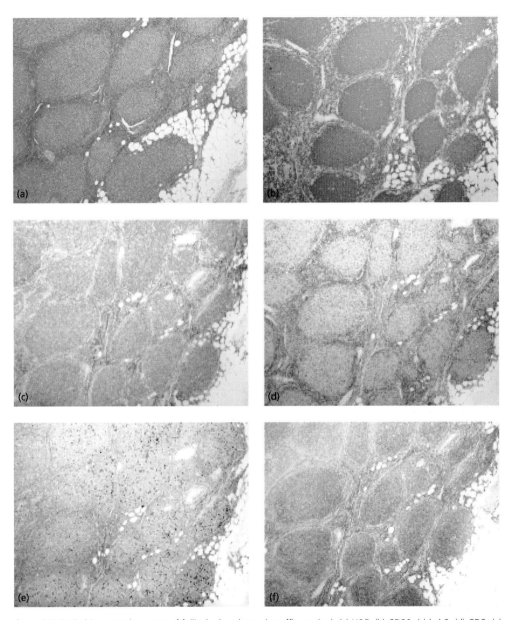

Figure 8.6 Typical immunophenotype of follicular lymphoma (paraffin section): (a) H&E, (b) CD20, (c) bcl-2, (d) CD3, (e) Ki67 and (f) CD10. *Source*: Courtesy of Professor Kevin Gatter.

Table 8.2 Staging of lymphomas.

Stage I	Involvement of a single lymph node group
Stage II	Involvement of two or more lymph node groups on one side of the diaphragm
Stage III	Involvement of lymph node groups on both sides of the diaphragm
Stage IV	Involvement of extralymphatic sites (e.g. bone marrow or liver)

Note: Patients are said to be symptom stage: (A) if they have no systemic symptoms, or symptom stage and (B) in the presence of any one of night sweats, fever, or weight loss (10% loss in past 6 months).

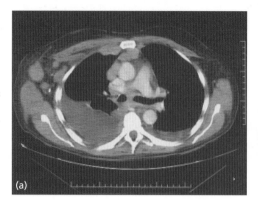 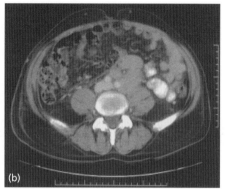

Figure 8.7 CT image of a lymphoma: (a) right axillary, anterior mediastinal nodal disease and bilateral pleural effusions and (b) bulky retroperitoneal lymphadenopathy (i.v. and bowel contrast help define the lymphomatous masses).

as the presence of a raised level is known to confer a poor prognosis. Immunoglobulins should be measured and monoclonal proteins looked for by immunoelectrophoresis.

Prognosis

The prognosis of non-Hodgkin lymphoma depends on the clinical entity; that is whether it is follicular, diffuse large B-cell lymphoma, Burkitt's, etc. However, for any of these lymphoma types there are a number of independent prognostic markers, the so-called international prognostic index (IPI) (Table 8.3 and Fig. 8.8).

Treatment and management

A number of different modalities are used in the treatment of lymphoma. Chemotherapy, radiotherapy, antibody treatment and bone marrow transplantation are all used either alone or in combination. Localized Hodgkin lymphoma and indolent lymphomas can be very effectively treated by radiotherapy. Widespread lymphomas require chemotherapy, either single or multiagent. Recently, a number of different antibodies against leucocyte-specific molecules have been developed for therapy. One such antibody (Rituximab) targets CD20 and has been found to have good activity in follicular and other lymphomas expressing this molecule (Fig. 8.9). Coupling these antibodies to radioactive isotopes appears to lead to improved response rates (e.g. ^{90}Y-labelled anti-CD20 antibodies). Restaging during treatment may guide the number of courses of chemotherapy. Staging CT scans are usually performed at the end of treatment to document the response — either complete remission (CR), partial remission (PR), or non-responders.

Table 8.3 The international prognostic index: features confering a worse prognosis.

Presence of extranodal disease: Disease outside lymphatic sites confers a poor prognosis
Advanced stage disease: Worse prognosis
Elevated LDH*: Worse prognosis
Performance status: Patients who are unable to care for themselves or are confined to bed have a worse prognosis
Age: Increasing age is associated with a poor prognosis

Note: * LDH — lactate dehydrogenase.

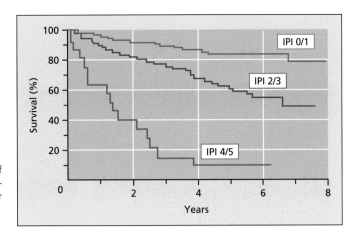

Figure 8.8 The overall survival of patients with follicular lymphoma sub-divided by the IPI score $p < 0.001$ for differences between the curves.

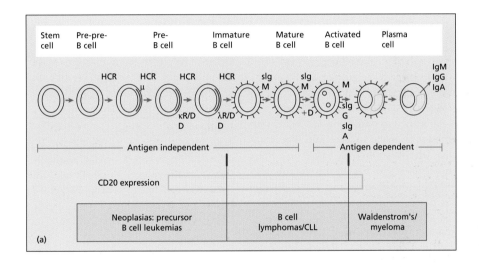

(a)

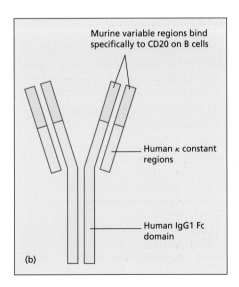

(b)

Figure 8.9 (a) The diagram shows the changes that occur during the maturation of a stem cell into plasma cells. Note that immature B cells and plasma cells do not express CD20. *Notes*: CLL — chronic lymphocytic leukaemia; HCR — heavy chain rearrangement; μ — mu heavy chain synthesis; κR/D — kappa chain rearrangement or deletion; λR/D — lambda chain rearrangement or deletion; sIgM, sIgG, sIgA — surface immunoglobulins M, G, and A, respectively. (b) A schematic diagram of Rituximab: a chimeric monoclonal antibody designed to bind to CD20 antigen on B cells inducing apoptosis and cell death.

Chapter 9

Classification of Lymphoma

Classification of lymphomas has been perceived as being complex and difficult. A successful classification must be useful in the clinic. The thrust of previous classifications was based on careful microscopy and relied heavily on morphology and limited immunophenotyping. The realization that there is a relationship between what is seen under the microscope and the clinical course of the patient has improved classification of human lymphoid neoplasms.

The so-called REAL classification of lympho–mas — a *r*evised *E*uropean–*A*merican classification of *l*ymphoid neoplasms was published in 1994 and has been modified to form the basis of the current World Health Organization (WHO) classification. Hodgkin lymphoma is divided into histological subtypes (Table 9.1, p. 100). The REAL/WHO classifications divide non-Hodgkin lymphomas into B-cell derived and T-cell derived neoplasms. Within these two broad divisions lie the clinico-pathological entities, that is tumours which derive from specific cell types and are associated

Table 9.1 Hodgkin lymphomas.

Classic	
Nodular sclerosing	The commonest type in young patients
Mixed cellularity	Second most common, may have worse prognosis
Lymphocyte deplete	
Lymphocyte rich	
Non-classic	
Lymphocyte-predominant	Behaves more like a low-grade non-Hodgkin lymphoma

with a predictable clinical picture (Tables 9.2, p. 101; Table 9.3, p. 101; Fig. 9.1, p. 102).

Unlike many of the former classifications, the REAL/WHO classification is useful to clinicians because it recognizes distinct lymphoma entities that may require specific treatment and management programmes. It is likely that within the current classification there will be additional entities not yet identified, which will be realized through a combination of immunophenotyping, cytogenetics and molecular analysis. The ability to look at differential gene expression using microarray technology may be of great value in this respect.

Lecture Notes: Haematology, by NC Hughes-Jones, SN Wickramsinghe, CSR Hatton © 2008 Blackwell Publishing, ISBN: 9781405180504

Table 9.2 Non-Hodgkin B-cell lymphomas.

Precursor B-cell neoplasms	
Precursor B-lymphoblastic leukaemia/lymphoma (ALL)	ALL is the commonest type of leukaemia found in children. Fatal if left untreated; needs multiagent chemotherapy with prophylactic CNS treatment to prevent CNS relapse
Peripheral B-cell neoplasms	
B-cell chronic lymphocytic leukaemia/small lymphocytic lymphoma (CLL/SLL)	CLL is the commonest type of leukaemia found in adults over 50 years. Presents with lymphocytosis, progresses to lymphadenopathy, hepatosplenomegaly and bone marrow failure. Treatment is usually with oral chemotherapy
B-cell prolymphocytic leukaemia	
Immunocytoma/Waldenstrom's macroglobulinemia (WM)	Indolent lymphoma presenting with bone marrow involvement, lymphadenopathy and hepatosplenomegaly. Typically has IgM paraprotein which may cause hyperviscosity or coagulation problems
Mantle cell lymphoma (MCL)	MCL presents with widespread lymphadenopathy, hepatosplenomegaly, bone marrow and extranodal (especially GI tract) involvement. Very poor prognosis
Follicle centre lymphoma (FCL)	Indolent lymphoma presenting with lymphadenopathy, bone marrow involvement and hepatosplenomegaly. High rate of transformation to large-cell lymphoma. Treatment with a combination of chemotherapy plus rituximab imparts the best outcome. Maintenance rituximab likely to be of benefit
Marginal zone B-cell lymphoma (includes MALT lymphomas and splenic lymphoma)	Usually extranodal lymphomas. The commonest mucosa-associated lymphoma affects the stomach. Often associated with *Helicobacter pylori* infection. May be widespread
Hairy cell leukaemia (HCL)	Presents with pancytopenia, circulating hairy cells and splenomegaly. Treatment with chemotherapy leads to sustained remissions
Plasmacytoma/myeloma	See Chapter 11
Diffuse large B-cell lymphoma (DLBC)	Aggressive and common lymphoma. Frequently presents with weight loss, fever, sweats and lymphadenopathy. Good response rates to a combination of rituximab and CHOP chemotherapy. Curable in 50% of cases
Burkitt lymphoma (BL)	Highly aggressive. Frequent extranodal involvement. Needs sequential multiagent chemotherapy

Table 9.3 Non-Hodgkin T-cell lymphomas.

Precursor T-cell neoplasm	
Precursor T-lymphoblastic leukaemia/lymphoma	T-cell ALL — for clinical picture, see B cell ALL above
Peripheral T-cell and NK-cell neoplasms	
T-cell prolymphocytic leukaemia	Rare, aggressive leukaemia responds poorly to chemotherapy. Better response rates to antibody therapy — Alemtuzumab
Large granular lymphocyte leukaemia (LGL)	Rare CD8+ indolent lymphoma associated with neutropenia
Mycosis fungoides, Sezary syndrome	Rare CD4+ lymphomas affecting the skin
Peripheral T-cell lymphomas, unspecified (PTC)	Widespread nodal disease associated with systemic symptoms — progress despite chemotherapy
Angioimmunoblastic T-cell lymphoma (AILD)	Rare aggressive lymphoma associated with fever, lymphadenopathy, skin rashes and Coomb's positive haemolytic anaemia. Poor prognosis
Enteropathy-associated-T-cell lymphoma (EATL)	Aggressive lymphoma associated with adult-onset coeliac disease
Adult T-cell lymphoma/leukaemia (ATL/L)	HTLV-1-associated lymphoma found with high prevalence in Japan, Caribbean and south-eastern USA. Usually very aggressive clinical course often complicated by hypercalcaemia. Many patients relapse in the CNS
Anaplastic large cell lymphoma (ALCL)	Occurs in childhood and young adults. Aggressive but many cases do well with combination chemotherapy

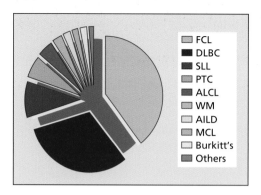

Figure 9.1 Pie chart showing the relative incidence of different non-Hodgkin lymphomas. For abbreviations see Tables 9.2 and 9.3.

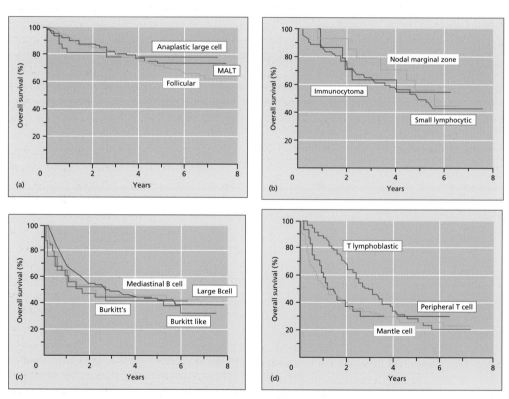

Figure 9.2 Survival curves for patients with different types of lymphoma. (a, b) Good prognosis lymphomas. (c, d) Poor prognosis lymphomas (note that mantle cell lymphoma (MCL) has the worst prognosis of any lymphoma).

Chapter 10

Neoplastic Disorders of Lymphoid Cells

Learning objectives

- To know the pathological changes, clinical presentation, investigation and principles of management of Hodgkin lymphoma.
- To know the pathological changes, clinical manifestations and the basic principles of treatment of the commoner non-Hodgkin lymphomas including acute lymphoblastic leukaemia (ALL), chronic lymphocytic leukaemia (CLL), diffuse large B-cell lymphoma (DLBC, high-grade lymphoma) and follicular lymphoma (low-grade lymphoma).

Hodgkin lymphoma

The first description of this disorder has been accredited to Dr. Thomas Hodgkin of Guy's Hospital following his account in 1832 of affected lymph glands in postmortem cases.

Hodgkin lymphoma is one of the commoner lymphomas seen in Western countries and is characterized by the presence of a low number of tumour cells designated Hodgkin's/Reed–Sternberg cells. The Reed–Sternberg cells are bi- or multinucleate, with each nucleus containing one prominent nucleolus. Other Hodgkin's cells are mononucleate.

Lecture Notes: Haematology, by NC Hughes-Jones, SN Wickramsinghe, CSR Hatton © 2008 Blackwell Publishing, ISBN: 9781405180504

The histological findings in a lymph node affected by Hodgkin lymphoma are scattered tumour cells admixed with reactive lymphocytes, plasma cells, macrophages, neutrophils, eosinophils and a variable amount of fibrosis. Under the term 'Hodgkin lymphoma' are recognized two clinically and biologically different entities: classic Hodgkin lymphoma, of which there are four histological types (Table 10.1), and non-classic Hodgkin lymphoma, which includes the entity of lymphocyte-predominant Hodgkin lymphoma (LPHL). Nodular sclerosis is the commonest histological subtype and is characterized by bands of fibrosis that enclose nodules of lymphoid tissue containing variable numbers of Hodgkin's cells (Fig. 10.1). Mixed cellularity is characterized by the presence of a heterogeneous mixture of lymphocytes, eosinophils, neutrophils, plasma cells, epithelial cells and Hodgkin's cells. In general, the more lymphocytes present the fewer the number of Hodgkin's cells and the better the prognosis. Lymphocyte-depleted Hodgkin lymphoma is a rare form and is characterized by a low number of lymphocytes, the absence of fibrous bands and by numerous, sometimes anaplastic, Hodgkin's/Reed–Sternberg cells. LPHL has a chronic relapsing course and often behaves more like follicular non-Hodgkin lymphoma (see below).

Whereas the B-cell nature of the tumour cells (called 'popcorn' cells or lymphocytic and histiocytic cells) of LPHL has been widely accepted, the cellular origin of the Reed–Sternberg cells of classic

Table 10.1 Rye classification of the histological appearances of lymph nodes in classic Hodgkin lymphoma.

Subgroup	Characteristics	Cases (%)	Surviving 5 years (%)
Lymphocyte rich	Infiltrate consists largely of small lymphocytes. There are only a few eosinophils, Reed–Sternberg cells and mononuclear Hodgkin's cells	15	70
Nodular sclerosing	The node is divided by broad bands of connective tissue into nodules containing a mixture of Reed–Sternberg cells, mononuclear Hodgkin's cells, lymphocytes, plasma cells, macrophages and eosinophils	40	60
Mixed cellularity	There are no broad bands of connective tissue. The node is diffusely infiltrated with the same mixture of cell types as above. Reed–Sternberg cells are readily seen. Fibrosis and focal necrosis are common	30	30
Lymphocyte depletion	Mononuclear Hodgkin's cells and Reed–Sternberg cells are present in large numbers. Relatively few lymphocytes are seen and there may be diffuse fibrosis	15	20

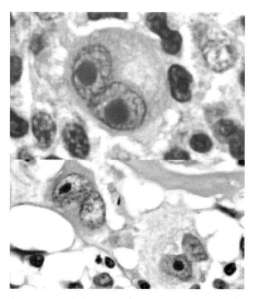

Figure 10.1 Photomicrograph showing Reed–Sternberg cells from a case of Hodgkin lymphoma.

Hodgkin lymphoma has been the subject of debate for many years. This was due to fact that although Reed–Sternberg cells express the lymphocyte-associated marker CD30, they do not consistently stain with markers for B or T cells. However, recent molecular techniques using single Reed–Sternberg cells microdissected from tissue sections have demonstrated that cells harbour clonal immunoglobulin gene rearrangements, thereby demonstrating Reed–Sternberg cells to be of B-cell origin.

Incidence and aetiology

Whereas the incidence of non-Hodgkin lymphoma has been increasing over the last 10–15 years, the incidence of Hodgkin lymphoma has remained stable at about 3 per 100,000 population; it is higher in men than in women. Hodgkin lymphoma increases in incidence with age, peaking in the third decade, followed by a decline. It used to be thought there was a second peak in later life but this has not been verified in recent studies. The nodular sclerosis type tends to occur in young adults.

The aetiology of Hodgkin lymphoma is unknown. The apparent geographical clustering of cases that has been reported has suggested an infectious aetiology and many efforts have been made to identify likely culprits. However, it seems that such clustering may have occurred by chance alone. Epstein–Barr virus (EBV) has long remained a favored possible cause because similar age groups are affected by both Hodgkin lymphoma and glandular fever. Indeed, there is some evidence that EBV might have a part to play in the aetiology of Hodgkin lymphoma, supported by the finding of clonal EBV DNA in 30–40% of cases.

Clinical features

The clinical features resemble those found in non-Hodgkin lymphoma. Lymph node enlargement

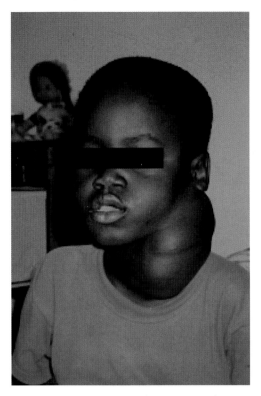

Figure 10.2 Massive cervical lymphadenopathy in a young boy with Hodgkin lymphoma.

Table 10.2 Basic features of the Ann Arbor staging system.

Stages	Characteristics
I	Involvement of one lymph node area
II	Involvement of two or more lymph node areas on the same side of the diaphragm
III	Involvement of lymph nodes on both sides of the diaphragm with or without involvement of the spleen
IV	Involvement of one or more extranodal sites (e.g. liver, marrow, lung)

Notes: A — without systemic symptoms; B — with systemic symptoms (night sweats, fever, weight loss).

Prognosis

A number of attempts have been made to predict outcome in patients treated for Hodgkin lymphoma. The prognosis is worse for males, older patients, patients with advanced disease and those patients with a low serum albumin concentration, anaemia and leukocytosis. Understanding prognostic factors may enable more intensive treatment to be given to patients with a predicted worse outcome, whilst those patients with a good prognosis could be spared unnecessary toxicity and adverse late effects.

Treatment

The goal of treatment for Hodgkin lymphoma is cure, whilst minimizing complications. Early-stage disease (stages IA–IIA) can be effectively treated with abbreviated chemotherapy together with localized radiotherapy. Patients who relapse can often be salvaged using combination chemotherapy or high-dose chemotherapy with peripheral blood stem-cell rescue.

Advanced disease (stages IIB–IV) is treated with six to eight courses of combination chemotherapy; radiotherapy is reserved to treat residual masses or given after completion of chemotherapy to areas previously involved by bulky disease. Modern treatment is based upon a number of considerations, most notably the need to attain a high cure rate, the need to minimize the toxicity of treatment and the need to preserve fertility. The high

is the commonest presentation, usually affecting the neck and mediastinum (Fig. 10.2). Spread is mainly along the lymph vessels; hence lymph node involvement tends to be contiguous. Sweats, fever, weight loss and pruritus may occur. Alcohol-induced pain in affected lymph nodes is thought to be virtually diagnostic. A not-infrequent presentation of Hodgkin lymphoma in young patients is cough, chest pain or dyspnoea as a result of extensive intrathoracic disease. Diagnosis is made by lymph node biopsy. The staging system using CT scanning is the same as that used for non-Hodgkin lymphoma (Table 10.2), except that the bone marrow is very rarely involved. A full blood count, erythrocyte sedimentation rate (ESR), liver function tests, renal and bone profile and lactate dehydrogenase (LDH) are all necessary and may confer prognostic information.

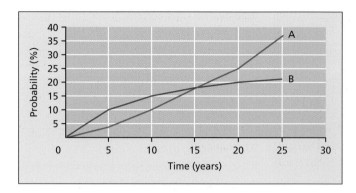

Figure 10.3 Actuarial risk of death from Hodgkin lymphoma (B) or other causes (A) in patients treated for Hodgkin lymphoma.

'cure' rate in Hodgkin lymphoma may be at the price of a higher death rate from second malignancies and other toxicities. Use of alkylating agents and radiotherapy is likely to contribute to this excess risk. This increase in death rate from 'non-Hodgkin' causes is graphically illustrated in Fig. 10.3. After 15 years from the diagnosis, the mortality from causes other than Hodgkin lymphoma is greater than deaths due to the lymphoma itself, though this trend may change as patients are treated with modern chemotherapy regimens which aim to reduce long-term toxicity. Irradiation of pubertal breast tissue is thought to put patients at particularly high risk of breast cancer.

Whilst early-stage Hodgkin lymphoma can be cured with radiotherapy, it was not until cyclical four-drug chemotherapy regimens such as MOPP were used in the late 1960s that advanced stage disease could be cured. MOPP (*m*ustine (alkylating agent), vincristine (*O*ncovin), *p*rednisolone and *p*rocarbazine), though very effective in at least half of all cases, has been found to be associated with secondary leukaemia (myelodysplasia and acute myeloblastic leukaemia) and a high incidence of infertility. Doxorubicin (Adriamycin) containing regimens (e.g. ABVD; Adriamycin, Bleomycin, Vinblastine, Dacarbazine) are favoured for initial treatment because of the low incidence of secondary leukaemia and the fact that most patients, both male and female, remain fertile. ABVD has been shown to be equally as effective as MOPP-like regimens. ABVD is myelosuppressive and two drugs of this four-drug regimen are associated with serious side effects: the use of

bleomycin can cause significant pulmonary toxicity and exposure to high doses of anthracyclines is known to cause cardiomyopathy. The latter two problems can be avoided by close monitoring and discontinuation of the drug that is responsible.

Patients who fail to respond to initial therapy, or who relapse, can be considered for high-dose therapy with peripheral blood stem-cell rescue. Approximately 40% of such patients respond well to this approach (see Chapter 13).

Positron emission tomography scanning

Positron emission tomography (*PET scanning*) may be useful to determine whether there is active disease in residual masses after the completion of therapy. The uptake of a radioactive fluorinated glucose molecule in active tumours may dictate whether further treatment such as radiotherapy is necessary. This technique is still under evaluation, but looks promising in both Hodgkin and non-Hodgkin lymphomas.

Non-Hodgkin lymphomas

Acute lymphoblastic leukaemia

Pathology

Lymphoblastic neoplasms of B-cell or T-cell type usually present as a leukaemia with circulating blast cells (acute lymphoblastic leukaemia, ALL); however, they may also present as a mediastinal mass with few circulating blast cells (the lymphoblastic lymphomas). In the leukaemia form, the marrow is heavily infiltrated with blast cells, which are also present in the peripheral blood (Fig. 10.4).

The disorder results from a clonal proliferation of cells from the earliest stages of lymphoid maturation (i.e. B or T blast cells). B-cell leukaemia blast cells have a phenotype defined by the presence of CD19, CD79a, CD10, CD34 and terminal deoxynucleotidyl transferase (TdT). T-cell markers such as CD7 and CD3 will define the cells as being of T-cell origin.

Cytogenetics

Cytogenetic analysis provides important prognostic information. Treatment regimens are increasingly based on risk stratification and, therefore, cytogenetics is an important part of the investigations at presentation. Hyperdiploidy (increased numbers of chromosomes beyond the diploid state) generally carries a good prognosis, whereas certain structural variants such as the presence of a Philadelphia chromosome t(9;22) are found in about 5% of children with ALL and this confers a very poor prognosis. Other poor prognostic findings include rearrangements of the *MLL* (mixed lineage leukaemia/lymphoma) gene and hypodiploidy.

Clinical and laboratory features

ALL is the commonest childhood cancer but may present at any age. In children, the peak incidence is between the ages of 2 and 4 years. The clinical manifestations are listed in Box 10.1, as are the laboratory findings. Most of the clinical manifestations can be explained in terms of bone marrow failure secondary to bone marrow infiltration.

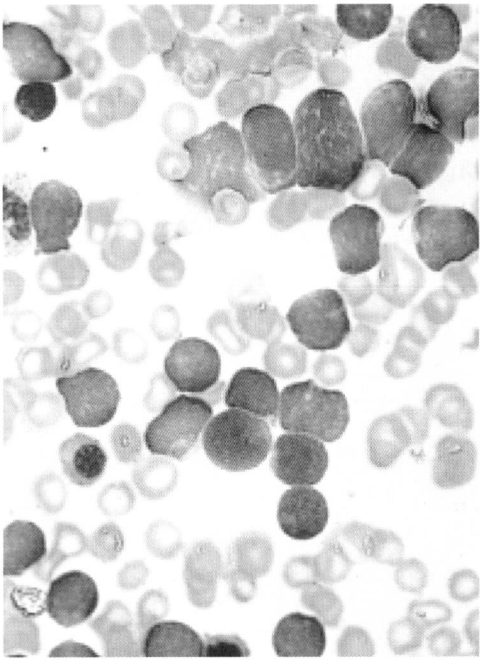

Figure 10.4 Bone marrow smear from a case of ALL. The blasts are small or medium-sized and have scanty cytoplasm. The nuclei have fine but densely-packed homogeneous-appearing chromatin and the nucleoli are small.

Box 10.1

Clinical features of ALL

Symptoms and their pathological basis
- Weakness, tiredness, malaise, lassitude
- Bruising and bleeding secondary to thrombocytopenia
- Otitis media, pharyngitis, pneumonia or fever due to bacterial infection caused by profound neutropenia
- Bone pain
- Enlarged lymph nodes
- Headache and vomiting resulting from CNS involvement leading to increased intracranial pressure

Physical findings
- Pallor
- Petechial haemorrhages, purpura and bruising
- Lymphadenopathy
- Hepatosplenomegaly
- Bone tenderness
- Fever

Laboratory features of ALL
- Anaemia
- Leukopenia
- Thrombocytopenia
- Blood film may show circulating blast cells
- Bone marrow usually heavily infiltrated with blast cells (>20%)

Treatment

Treatment of childhood acute leukaemia has improved greatly, due largely to the results of clinical trials that have been conducted over the last 20–30 years. Risk stratification based on prognostic factors is used to determine the protocols on which children and adults with ALL are treated, though the general schema is outlined below. The treatment is by chemotherapy, given in four phases:

1 *Induction*: The aim of induction chemotherapy is to clear the bone marrow of leukaemia blast cells and replace them with normal hemopoietic cells.
2 *Consolidation*: Consolidation therapy reduces the leukaemia cell burden further and uses a combination of moderately intensive treatment after normal hemopoiesis has been restored with induction chemotherapy.
3 *CNS prophylaxis*: A phase of prophylactic treatment to prevent central nervous system involvement is always given. This can be achieved by the administration of high-dose chemotherapy drugs such as methotrexate which cross the blood–brain barrier, or by direct administration of drugs into the cerebrospinal fluid (intrathecal), or by giving external beam radiotherapy.
4 *Maintenance therapy*: The final treatment phase is that of maintenance therapy. Continuous oral and intermittent intravenous chemotherapy is given over 2–3 years.

Prognosis

A number of prognostic factors determine outcome in ALL. Boys do worse than girls and a high white cell count at presentation and an age over 10 years also confer a poor prognosis. Low-risk childhood ALL can be cured in a high percentage of cases. Patients who relapse or who present in the poorest risk categories should be considered for allogeneic bone marrow transplantation (Chapter 13). Adults with ALL do not have such a good prognosis and may be offered allogeneic bone marrow transplantation in the first remission.

Lymphoblastic lymphoma

This represents the lymphomatous equivalent of ALL (i.e. there is little peripheral blood or bone marrow involvement). It has very similar features to ALL but there are a number of characteristic clinical features: it is commoner in adolescent males and it frequently presents with a mediastinal mass. Patients must have less than 20% blasts in their bone marrow otherwise they are classified as having ALL. Lymphoblastic lymphoma is treated using the same protocols as for ALL.

B-cell chronic lymphocytic leukaemia

Chronic lymphocytic leukaemia (CLL) is a neoplastic disorder characterized by the accumulation of small mature lymphocytes in the blood (Fig. 10.5), bone marrow and lymphoid tissues. This is the commonest leukaemia seen in the Western world, and tends to affect almost exclusively adults over the age of 50 years. The cells which give rise to the disorder express the B-cell markers CD19 and CD20. They also express CD23, are negative for CD10, but express the T-cell marker CD5 and weakly express surface IgM. Cytogenetic studies confer some prognostic information: for example, deletions involving chromosome 17 (p53 deletions) confer a very poor prognosis. The clinical and laboratory features of CLL are summarized in Box 10.2.

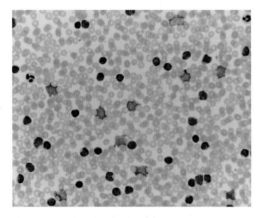

Figure 10.5 Blood film in a patient with B-cell CLL. Note the presence of increased numbers of small lymphocytes and some smear cells.

Box 10.2

Clinical features of CLL

Symptoms and their pathological basis
- Most patients are over 60 years of age
- Many patients are asymptomatic at diagnosis
- Patients may present with symptoms attributable to anaemia — tiredness and fatigue
- Bruising and bleeding secondary to thrombocytopenia
- Sinusitis, bacterial pneumonia — secondary to hypogammaglobulinaemia
- Night sweats, fever and weight loss are uncommon but may occur

Physical findings
- Lymphadenopathy
- Hepatosplenomegaly

Laboratory features of CLL
- Monoclonal lymphocytosis is greater than 5×10^9/L
- In the more advanced stages of the disease there may be anaemia and thrombocytopenia
- The direct antiglobulin (Coomb's) test may be positive
- Bone marrow aspirate and trephine biopsy demonstrates the extent of bone marrow infiltration
- Hypogammaglobulinaemia is a common finding — a small proportion of patients will have a monoclonal band on immunoelectrophoresis
- Immunophenotyping of the malignant lymphocytes show expression of CD5, CD19, CD20, CD23 and CD79a and surface IgM (weakly positive); CD10 is negative

Autoimmune phenomena may occur in patients with CLL. The most common manifestations are autoimmune haemolytic anaemia (AIHA) and autoimmune thrombocytopenic purpura (ITP). Patients may rarely develop pure red cell aplasia or neutropenia. Acquired angioneurotic oedema may also result from autoimmune antibodies against the C1 esterase inhibitor. The antibodies are not thought to be produced by the malignant B cells but rather by bystander populations of normal B cells.

CLL has a predictable natural history. Most patients have only a lymphocytosis at the beginning of their illness and progress to develop lymphadenopathy, hepatosplenomegaly and finally bone marrow failure. It is the presence or absence of these features which determine the prognosis.

Hypogammaglobulinaemia

Patients with CLL commonly have an associated hypogammaglobulinaemia. A reduction in the serum levels of IgM, IgG and IgA may all occur and these predispose to infections, particularly of the respiratory tract, by capsulated organisms such as *Steptococcus pneumoniae* and *Haemophilus influenzae*.

Small lymphocytic B-cell lymphoma

Small lymphocytic lymphoma (SLL) is the lymphomatous equivalent of CLL without abnormal cells in the peripheral blood, and has the same biology and clinical features. The disease is characterized by lymph node involvement and bone marrow infiltration.

Treatment of CLL/SLL

Patients with CLL/SLL who are asymptomatic often do not require treatment; simple monitoring in the clinic is sufficient. Indications for treatment include systemic symptoms such as sweats, fever, weight loss or cytopenias such as anaemia. Many elderly patients with progressive disease can be safely treated with a simple regimen of oral chlorambucil. For younger patients oral chlorambucil is still a useful agent but higher responses can be obtained with fludarabine or a combination of fludarabine and cyclophosphamide. No survival advantage for these more aggressive chemotherapy regimens has been demonstrated so it is uncertain whether higher response rates or indeed improved duration of response is a definite advantage. Indeed, combination chemotherapy may lead to an increase in infection rates and lead to greater overall toxicity. Furthermore, the addition of antibodies designed to target antigens expressed on B cells, such as the anti-CD20 antibody Rituximab, may increase the response rate still further. Trials are underway to find out whether combination chemotherapy alongside targeted antibody therapy will improve overall survival. Other treatments are sometimes used, including multiagent chemotherapy such as CHOP in high-grade transformation and Campath antibody therapy in patients with chemorefractory disease. The median survival of all patients with B-cell CLL is 10–12 years. More intensive treatment including bone marrow transplantation is sometimes attempted in younger patients.

Waldenström's macroglobulinaemia

This disorder usually behaves in a low-grade fashion. Like CLL this is a disease found in patients who are in their sixth or seventh decade. The malignant cells are fairly mature B cells capable of secreting IgM. The bone marrow is typically involved, as are the liver and spleen. Lymphadenopathy is also a common feature. The disorder can be dominated by clinical manifestations consequent upon high levels of monoclonal IgM; the condition is then known as Waldenström's macroglobulinaemia.

High concentrations of IgM and the accompanying hyperviscosity cause headache, visual disturbances (fundoscopic examination may reveal dilated veins, papilledema and retinal haemorrhage) and altered consciousness. There may also be bleeding or thrombosis.

The IgM paraprotein may have unusual physical properties such as causing red cell agglutination (cold agglutinins) or precipitating in cold temperatures (cryoglobulin).

Patients are frequently anaemic and experience symptoms of tiredness and fatigue. The fatigue is often out of proportion to the level of haemoglobin. Systemic symptoms such as fever, weight loss and night sweats may occur, particularly if the lymphoma undergoes high-grade transformation.

Laboratory findings are summarized in Table 10.3.

Table 10.3 Laboratory findings in Waldenstroms Macroglobulinaemia.

Anaemia
Leukopenia
Thrombocytopenia
Lymphocytosis may occur
IgM monoclonal protein
Bone marrow infiltration with lymphoid cells

Treatment

Single-agent oral chlorambucil is the first line of therapy. Patients who fail to respond to chlorambucil can be treated with fludarabine, or combinations or fludarabine and cyclophosphamide. The addition of rituximab may increase response rates. Combination chemotherapy such as CHOP can be useful, particularly if there is high-grade transformation. Hyperviscosity syndrome requires urgent plasma exchange.

The immunophenotype is CD20+, CD19+, CD5−, sIg+ and CD10−.

Follicular lymphoma

Follicular lymphoma is relatively easy for the pathologist to identify because of its follicular growth pattern (see Fig. 8,6). The disorder typifies the so-called low-grade lymphomas, being indolent in its clinical course but remaining incurable. Follicular lymphoma is associated with a translocation between chromosome 14 and 18 t(14;18), which leads to the upregulation of the anti-apoptotic protein BCL-2.

This is one of the commonest types of lymphoma. Most patients present with widespread lymphadenopathy, bone marrow infiltration and hepatosplenomegaly. Occasionally this lymphoma may present in an extranodal fashion, the gastrointestinal tract and the skin being among the more usual sites of involvement.

The clinical course alternates between stable periods when patients remain well and periods of progressive disease requiring therapy. High-grade transformation in which there is development of large cell lymphoma (see below) occurs in 60% of patients, but with combination chemotherapy patients can be 'cured of the high-grade component' and revert to having low-grade lymphoma. Nevertheless, high-grade transformation confers a poor prognosis.

There is no evidence that early or intensive treatment of follicular lymphoma at presentation improves outcome. Therapy is required, however, in patients with systemic symptoms, critical organ failure or bulky disease. Randomized controlled trials have shown a survival advantage for the addition of the anti-CD20 antibody rituximab(R) to commonly used first-line chemotherapy regimens such as cyclophosphamide, vincristine and prednisolone (CVP). Patients who relapse after first-line chemotherapy can often be effectively treated with regimens such as R-CHOP or regimens containing fludarabine. Furthermore, there is now increasing evidence to suggest that maintenance rituximab may benefit those patients who have a good response to second-line chemotherapy. Studies are underway to determine whether maintenance rituximab will also benefit patients after first-line chemotherapy.

Patients who respond well to second-line treatment and who are otherwise fit can be considered for more intensive, perhaps even curative, strategies such as high-dose therapy and stem-cell rescue or reduced-intensity conditioning (RIC) allografting. Older patients can be treated with the single oral alkylating agent chlorambucil, with or without rituximab.

Low-grade lymphomas are often extremely radiosensitive and radiotherapy can be useful for treating localized or bulky disease. An alternative approach involves conjugating a β-emitting radioisotope to an anti-CD20 antibody. This allows the delivery of radiation directly to the site of disease. This strategy has been shown to be an effective therapy for patients with follicular lymphoma and may be incorporated into future treatment strategies. In addition, other radioisotopes, including γ-emitters, have been linked with anti-CD20 antibodes with the same aim.

The prognosis of follicular lymphoma is variable and is anything from 2 to 20 years. The median survival is about 10–12 years from diagnosis.

The immunophenotype is CD19+e, CD20+, CD10+, BCL-2+ and BCL-6+.

Mantle cell lymphoma

Mantle cell lymphoma is an aggressive low-grade lymphoma. This lymphoma entity is commoner in males and generally presents in older patients with a median age of 60 years. The malignant cells are thought to derive from cells of the mantle zone of the lymph node follicle

(Fig. 10.6(a)). The lymphoma cells are small to medium sized and in common with CLL express CD5. In contrast to CLL, mantle cell lymphoma does not express CD23 and there is a characteristic cytogenetic abnormality that is found in a high proportion of cases. A translocation between chromosome 11 and chromosome 14 t(11;14), leads to the upregulation of the protein cyclin D1, which is known to play a key role in cell cycle regulation (Fig. 10.6(b)).

The disorder presents with widespread lymphadenopathy, hepatosplenomegaly and bone marrow involvement and often abnormal lymphocytes can be seen in the peripheral blood. Some series have reported a very high incidence of gastrointestinal involvement (>80%). Systemic symptoms are unusual, most patients feeling reasonably well at the time of presentation. The disease runs an aggressive course with a mean survival of 2–4 years. The disorder is not curable and though intensive chemotherapy is often given, there is no very effective therapy. For those patients with aggressive disease and who have responded to chemotherapy, experimental treatment with high-dose therapy or RIC allograft should be considered.

The immunophenotype is CD19+, CD20+, CD5+, CD23−, IgM+ and cyclin D1+.

Hairy cell leukaemia

This uncommon disorder frequently affects middle-aged males. It typically presents with pancytopenia and splenomegaly. Characteristic hairy cells are usually found on examination of a peripheral blood film (Fig. 10.7). The disorder is diagnosed by microscopy of the blood and bone marrow examination. Immunophenotyping and cytochemistry help to define the disorder.

Hairy cell leukaemia behaves in an indolent manner, responds well to treatment with single-agent drugs such as 2-chlorodeoxyadenosine (cladribine) or pentostatin. Splenectomy and α-interferon are also effective treatment strategies.

The immunophenotype is CD23−, CD5−, Ig+, CD25+ and CD11c+.

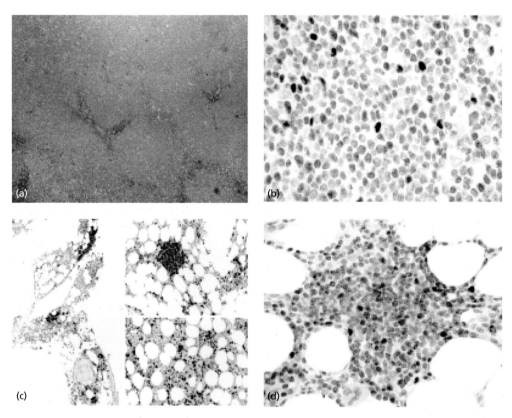

Figure 10.6 (a) The non-specific histological appearance seen in the biopsy of a patient with mantle cell lymphoma; (b) staining using an antibody against cyclin D1 which is overexpressed in mantle cell lymphoma; (c) minimal disease after treatment identified by cyclin D1 staining; and (d) high-power view.

Diffuse large B-cell lymphoma

Diffuse large B-cell lymphoma (DLBC) is the commonest high-grade lymphoma. It typifies an aggressive but potentially curable lymphoma, and represents approximately one-third of all lymphomas. Histologically, the disorder is characterized by the presence of large cells of B-cell origin. The disorder probably includes a variety of different lymphoma types and in this sense is a bit of a dustbin for those lymphomas that do not obviously fit into other categories. Microarray technology has identified at least two different types of DLBC based on gene expression profiling.

The disorder occurs at all ages but becomes commoner in later life. Patients may present with night sweats, fever, weight loss and lymphadenopathy or with extranodal lymphoma involving sites such as the gastrointestinal tract, the testis, brain or bone. Treatment is with combination chemotherapy which can induce remission in approximately 80% of cases, though only 30–40% of patients will attain a sustained remission beyond 3 years. The combination of cyclophosphamide, doxorubicin (*h*ydroxydaunorubicin), vincristine (Oncovin) and *p*rednisolone (CHOP) has been the gold standard against which other treatments are judged. The treatment is administered every 3 weeks for a total of six or eight courses on an outpatient basis. The addition of the anti-CD20 antibody Rituximab to CHOP chemotherapy has improved survival rates so that the combination of rituximab and CHOP (R-CHOP) has become the standard of care for patients with DLBC lymphoma. This finding is particularly significant for those patients with low-risk disease (Fig. 10.8).

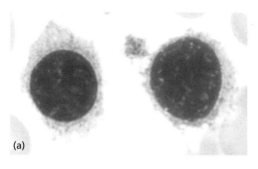

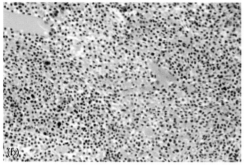

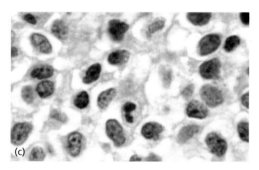

Figure 10.7 (a) Photomicrograph showing hairy cells in peripheral blood; (b) low power view of trephine biopsy showing infiltration and hemorrhage; and (c) high-power view of trephine biopsy. The hairy cells have bean-shaped nuclei and abundant empty-looking cytoplasm (appearing like a halo around the nucleus).

Relapsed patients can be offered high-dose chemotherapy and peripheral blood stem-cell rescue (Chapter 13). Patients who have chemo-sensitive disease may benefit from this approach. Radiotherapy is often given to sites of bulky disease or residual masses after the completion of chemotherapy.

The immunophenotype is CD20+, CD79+, CD5−, CD23−, CD10− and sIgM+.

Mucosa-associated lymphoid tissue lymphomas

The so-called mucosa-associated lymphoid tissue (MALT) lymphomas are typically extranodal as their name suggests. This type of lymphoma belongs to the group of marginal zone lymphomas as the malignant cells are thought to derive from the marginal zone of the lymphoid follicle. The commonest type is gastric MALT lymphoma. Patients usually present with a long history of indigestion and are found to have MALT lymphoma on gastric biopsy. Some, but by no means all, are associated with the presence of *Helicobater pylori*. Eradication of the bacterium using combination antibiotic therapy often leads to eradication of the lymphoma. In those cases that cannot be treated successfully with antibiotics, gentle oral chemotherapy or involved radiotherapy will usually control the disease. High-grade transformation may occur and is treated in the usual way with combination chemotherapy. Other common sites to be involved with this lymphoma include the thyroid gland, salivary glands, the lungs and the spleen.

The immunophenotype is CD20+, CD79+, CD5−, CD23−, CD10− and sIgM+.

AIDS-related lymphoma

Lymphoma is an AIDS-defining illness. Patients infected with HIV have a substantially increased risk of having lymphoma compared to the general population. The use of antiretroviral therapy has led to a decline in the incidence of AIDS-related non-Hodgkin lymphoma.

AIDS lymphoma is nearly always a B-cell neoplasm, most commonly of Burkitt's or diffuse large B-cell type. There is a propensity for involvement of extranodal sites, such as the gastrointestinal tract or the brain. Primary CNS lymphoma is a very rare finding in non-HIV-infected persons and HIV infection should be suspected in all such cases. AIDS-related lymphoma is a very aggressive disorder and the prognosis is generally poor. The use of antiretroviral therapy and combination chemotherapy has been reported to improve the prognosis.

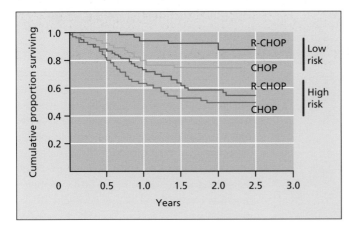

Figure 10.8 The survival of patients with DLBC lymphoma following treatment with CHOP alone compared with CHOP plus Rituximab (R-CHOP). Note the survival difference is more pronounced for patients with low-risk disease.

Mycosis fungoides and Sezary syndrome

These disorders are T-cell cutaneous lymphomas. Mycosis fungoides is an indolent disorder characterized by plaques or nodules affecting the skin. The disorder can be controlled with PUVA, and often waxes and wanes over many years. The disorder may eventually become systemic, and when this happens the prognosis is very poor. Sezary syndrome is characterized by generalized erythroderma and circulating abnormal lymphoid cells with cerebriform nuclei (Sezary cells) in the peripheral blood.

Chapter 11

Myeloma and Other Paraproteinaemias

Learning objectives

• To understand the meaning of the term 'paraprotein' and to know the various clinical situations in which a paraprotein may be found.
• To have a moderately detailed knowledge of the pathology, clinical features and diagnosis of myeloma and to understand the principles of treatment of this disorder.

Multiple myeloma

Multiple myeloma is a disease arising from the malignant transformation of a B cell or, possibly, a pre-B cell or earlier cell. The differentiating cells of the malignant clone have the morphology of plasma cells or plasmacytoid lymphocytes, have clonally rearranged immunoglobulin genes (see pp. 87–89), and usually secrete a monoclonal immunoglobulin, IgG or IgA, a monoclonal light chain, or both. Such monoclonal proteins are called paraproteins; they consist of structurally identical molecules and therefore produce a discrete band (M band) on electrophoresis. The primary site of proliferation of the malignant cells is the bone marrow, which shows many nodules of tumour tissue as well as diffuse interstitial infiltration (Fig. 11.1).

Lecture Notes: Haematology, by NC Hughes-Jones, SN Wickramsinghe, CSR Hatton © 2008 Blackwell Publishing, ISBN: 9781405180504

Activation of osteoclasts by molecules secreted from stromal cells and possibly the myeloma cells themselves, causes bone destruction that leads to multiple well-defined osteolytic lesions, radiological changes resembling those of generalized osteoporosis and hypercalcaemia. Marrow infiltration also causes impairment of haemopoiesis and haematological abnormalities. Some patients with IgA paraproteins (which tend to polymerize) and a few patients with high levels of IgG3 paraproteins have a substantially raised plasma viscosity and may suffer from the hyperviscosity syndrome. Light chains are filtered through the glomeruli and are found in the urine; they may eventually damage the renal tubules. In 10% of patients, the paraprotein is converted into deposits of amyloid in various tissues. Levels of normal Ig are reduced and in advanced disease there is a reduction in circulating T cells. Extramedullary tumour deposits develop frequently.

Clinical features

The incidence of myeloma is about 40 per million of the population per year. Thus, approximately 2500 new cases are diagnosed each year. Most patients are between the ages of 50 and 70 years. In some cases there is a prolonged asymptomatic phase which may last for a number of years — so-called monoclonal gammopathy of undetermined significance (MGUS). As the disease

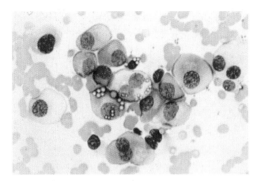

Figure 11.1 A marrow smear from a patient with multiple myeloma (May–Grünwald–Giemsa (MGG) stain).

advances and the bone marrow becomes infiltrated with malignant plasma cells secreting monoclonal immunoglobulin, a number of secondary changes may be found.

Bone destruction

The most common presenting symptom is bone pain, usually over the lumbar spine. Pathological fractures are frequent and often affect the lower thoracic and upper lumbar vertebrae and the ribs (Fig. 11.2). Compression fractures of the vertebrae may damage the spinal cord or spinal roots and cause neurological symptoms. Large tumours may form in relation to any bone and cause pressure symptoms.

Renal failure

Renal failure may be found at presentation or develop during the course of the disease. Chronic renal failure commonly results from the obstruction of distal renal tubules by proteinaceous casts leading to tubular atrophy and interstitial fibrosis (myeloma kidney). Renal dysfunction may also result from the toxic effects of light chains on tubule cells, the deposition of light chains in glomeruli and amyloidosis. Acute renal failure may be precipitated by dehydration, or be caused by hypercalcaemia or hyperuricaemia.

Bone marrow failure

Anaemia, neutropenia and thrombocytopenia may occur. The anaemia is usually normocytic or

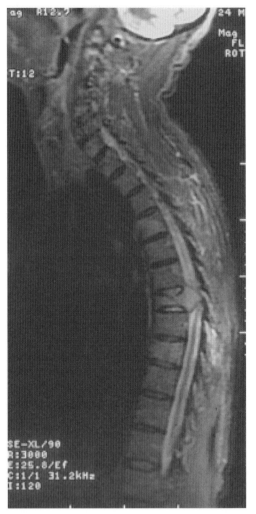

Figure 11.2 MRI of the spine showing spinal cord compression secondary to myeloma.

macrocytic. Mucosal bleeding is a common symptom and is due to interference with fibrin polymerization and platelet function. Platelet counts may be low in advanced cases.

Bacterial infections

Respiratory tract infections are common in patients with myeloma. The lack of normal antibodies (acquired hypogammaglobulinaemia) results in infections caused by capsulated organisms, commonly pneumococcus and haemophilus.

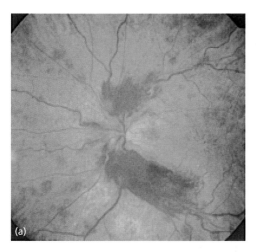 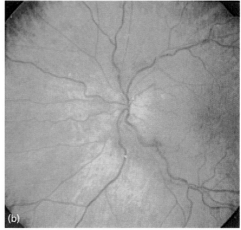

Figure 11.3 Fundi of the eyes in the hyperviscosity syndrome showing retinal haemorrhages (a) and papilloedema (b).

Thus, pneumonia and sinusitis are common presentations.

Hypercalcaemia

Hypercalcaemia causes symptoms such as anorexia, vomiting, lethargy, stupor or coma. Patients may present more acutely with polyuria and polydipsia.

Amyloidosis

Peripheral neuropathy, macroglossia, cardiomegaly, diarrhoea and carpal tunnel syndrome suggest amyloidosis. Peripheral neuropathy may also be caused by infiltration of nerves by plasma cells or by a direct toxic effect of the paraprotein.

Hyperviscosity syndrome

This is characterized by neurological disturbances (dizziness, somnolence and coma), cardiac failure and haemorrhagic manifestations (Fig. 11.3). IgA myeloma is more likely to cause hyperviscosity as IgA has a tendency to form dimers.

Laboratory findings

A normochromic, normocytic or macrocytic anaemia is common. When the disease is advanced, thrombocytopenia and neutropenia may also be found. The blood film may show a leucoerythroblastic picture and occasional plasma cells; red

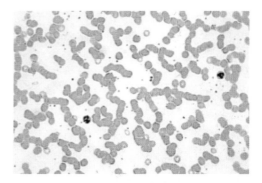

Figure 11.4 Blood film from a patient with multiple myeloma showing marked red cell rouleaux formation (MGG stain).

cells may show an increased tendency to form rouleaux (Fig. 11.4) and the paraprotein may cause an increased basophilic staining of the background in between the red cells. The erythrocyte sedimentation rate (ESR) is often raised, sometimes to more than 100 mm/h. The serum uric acid is raised in about half the cases (and may contribute to the renal damage).

Bone marrow aspirates usually contain a greatly increased proportion of plasma cells (Figs 11.1 and 11.5(a)). The latter may either appear normal or show various atypical features such as marked pleomorphism, pronounced multinuclearity, immaturity of the nucleus (i.e. finely distributed chromatin and nucleoli) and dissociation

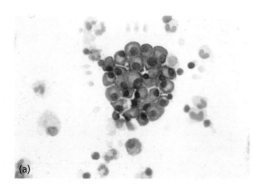
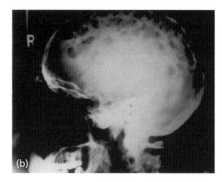

Figure 11.5 (a) Marrow smear showing myeloma cells reacting with antibody against λ-chains; the reaction was demonstrated using an immunoalkaline phosphatase method. The cells did not react with antibody against κ-chains and were therefore monoclonal in origin. The serum contained an IgD λ paraprotein. (b) Radiograph of the skull of a patient with multiple myeloma showing multiple discrete osteolytic lesions with no sclerosis at the margin.

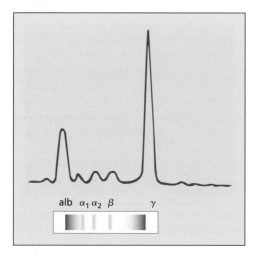

Figure 11.6 Illustration of serum electrophoresis demonstrating a monoclonal band and reduced normal immunoglobulins. *Source*: Courtesy of Professor Hoffbrand.

Light chains (also called Bence-Jones proteins) can be detected in the serum using the sensitive 'free lite assay' though it should be remembered that the vast majority of light chains are filtered by the kidney into the urine. They can be measured in urine and are best detected and studied by electrophoresis and immunofixation. Conversely, whole Ig molecules only appear in the urine when there is renal damage. In 50% of patients with myeloma, the paraprotein is IgG, in 25% it is IgA, in 20% it is light chain only, and in 1–2% it is IgD or IgE. IgM-producing myelomas are extremely rare. Over half the patients with an IgG- or IgA-secreting myeloma have monoclonal light chains in their urine; in two-thirds of these patients the light chain is κ and in the remainder it is λ. In 1–2% of patients with myeloma, paraprotein cannot be detected in either serum or concentrated urine (non-secretory myeloma).

Serum levels of β_2-microglobulin (the light chain of the HLA class 1 glycoproteins) correlates with tumour mass and together with the serum albumin is a very important prognostic marker (see below).

between nuclear and cytoplasmic maturation. Some aspirates may show only a slight increase in plasma cells (5–10% of nucleated marrow cells as compared with 0.1–2% in normal marrow) and others may show no increase. The latter results from the multifocal nature of the plasma cell infiltrate.

Electrophoresis of serum usually demonstrates the monoclonal Ig as a discrete band (M band) (Fig. 11.6) and the nature of the paraprotein can be determined by immunofixation. Each Ig class may be quantified using rate immunonephelometry.

Diagnosis

This is often based on the finding of at least two of the following three features:

1 A monoclonal Ig in the serum or monoclonal light chains in the urine or both.

2 An increased proportion of plasma cells (often with atypical features) in marrow aspirates.

3 Discrete osteolytic lesions on X-ray studies (Fig. 11.5(b)).

The differential diagnosis is from a benign paraproteinaemia (p. 120).

Treatment

Treatment should be reserved for patients with signs of progressive disease. Some patients may fulfil the criteria of myeloma but have indolent or smouldering disease with stable paraproteins and an absence of lytic bone lesions. Treatment requires a multidisciplinary approach involving haematologists/oncologists, nurse specialists, radiology, renal physicians, neurosurgeons, orthopaedic surgeons and palliative care specialists.

Supportive care measures are very important. Anaemia is commonly present as an integral component of the disease itself or secondary to treatment, and patients who require frequent transfusion may benefit from subcutaneous erythropoietin. Adequate hydration and a good urine flow must be maintained in an attempt to reduce the risk of paraprotein precipitation in the renal tubules and consequent renal damage; haemodialysis may be required in the event of renal failure. Patients with high paraprotein levels may also develop the hyperviscosity syndrome and plasma exchange can be used to rapidly reduce the effect of this problem. Bacterial infections require prompt treatment with antibiotics. Bone pain and fractures and hypercalcaemia cause significant morbidity and mortality in patients with myeloma. Long-term therapy with bisphosphonates has been shown to reduce bone pain and progression of skeletal lesions.

Chemotherapy

Cytotoxic drugs are usually reserved for patients with extensive or symptomatic bone lesions, hypercalcaemia, bone marrow failure, substantial Bence-Jones proteinuria or any renal dysfunction. Patients over 70 years are usually treated with melphalan or cyclophosphamide given orally with or without prednisolone, either intermittently (for 4–5 days every 4 weeks) or in smaller doses, continuously. Recently, the addition of thalidomide has been shown to increase the response rate and the combination of melphalan, prednisolone and thalidomide (MPT) has become the standard of care for older patients who are eligible for treatment. The mechanism of action of thalidomide is unknown but there is evidence to suggest that it may have antiangiogenic effects in myeloma. However, it has a number of troublesome side effects including drowsiness, constipation and peripheral neuropathy in addition to its well-known teratogenicity.

Approximately 75–80% of patients respond to MPT, with an improvement in symptoms, a rise in haemoglobin and a reduction in the paraprotein level. The response is gradual and may take many months. Treatment reduces the tumour mass and is usually stopped when the paraprotein level ceases to fall (plateau phase).

In younger patients, chemotherapy programmes are undergoing a period of revision. Vincristine, adriamycin and dexamethasone (VAD) used to be the first line therapy for this aggressive disease in most centres. However, combinations of thalidomide or its analogues (lenalidamide) combined with cyclophosphamide or dexamethasone or both (e.g. CTD) are being increasingly used as front-line treatment. Response rates have been found to be very high though it remains to be seen whether these responses will be durable. Following first line therapy, stem cells may be harvested and the patient treated with high-dose melphalan (200 mg/m^2) and peripheral stem cell rescue (Chapter 13). This treatment is not curative with over 90% of patients relapsing, but may give patients an additional few years of good quality life free of therapy.

Radiotherapy

Radiotherapy is a very effective treatment for bone pain in myeloma. Spinal cord compression due to a vertebral or a paravertebral mass requires urgent assessment, and decompression laminectomy followed by radiotherapy is usually the treatment of choice. Bone fractures, which are a common complication, are best treated by orthopaedic fixation followed by radiotherapy.

Relapsed and refractory disease

Nearly all patients with myeloma will relapse after the initial therapy. Occasional patients have been cured with allogeneic bone marrow transplantation but the technique is only suitable for patients under 45 years and carries a high mortality (Chapter 13). New agents continue to be developed for the treatment of relapsed myeloma. Bortezomib is a novel drug that inhibits the activity of the proteasome, the organelle responsible for regulated intracellular proteolysis. This agent has shown responses in 30–40% of patients with relapsed myeloma probably by preventing the degradation of IκB by the proteasome. IκB neutralizes NFκB, a molecule that drives cell proliferation.

Other treatment options for relapsed myeloma include the use of the thalidomide analogue lenalidomide, or the oral alkylating agent melphalan. Palliative care services need to be involved for expert advice on pain control and management of specific symptoms.

Prognosis

The median survival from diagnosis is 3–5 years. Patients presenting with anaemia or renal failure have a worse prognosis. Patients can be stratified according to the levels of serum β_2-microglobulin (a reflection of tumour burden and renal function) and albumin levels. High levels of β_2-microglobulin and low levels of albumin confer a poor prognosis. Certain cytogenetic abnormalities also provide prognostic information. Patients with deletions or partial deletions of chromosome 13 have a significantly worse outcome.

Solitary plasmacytoma

Solitary tumours consisting of malignant plasma cells may be found in the bone marrow or in extramedullary sites such as the upper respiratory tract. It is common to find a monoclonal Ig in the serum or monoclonal light chains in the urine, or both. In the case of extramedullary plasmacytomas, there is often no evidence of tumour elsewhere and the prognosis after excision followed by local radiotherapy is very good.

Other paraproteinaemias and related disorders

Benign paraproteinaemia (benign monoclonal gammopathy or monoclonal gammopathy of undetermined significance, MGUS)

A paraprotein is found in the serum in 0.1–1.0% of normal adults and in up to 10% of elderly subjects. A high proportion of such individuals suffer from a condition termed 'benign paraproteinaemia' that does not require treatment. The most important difference between MGUS and myeloma is the absence of end organ damage in the former. However, MGUS will transform to myeloma at the rate of 1% per year, emphasizing the importance of monitoring patients with an apparently benign paraproteinaemia. The differences between myeloma and MGUS are illustrated in Table 11.1.

Amyloidosis

Amyloidosis is a disorder of protein folding whereby normally soluble proteins are deposited as β-pleated sheets. Infiltration of organs with amyloid leads to dysfunction and eventual organ failure. Amyloid may be demonstrated in rectal, gingival or renal biopsies; it stains positively with Congo red and shows an apple green birefringence in polarized light. Amyloid may be of three principal types:

1 *AA amyloid*: Seen in patients with long-term chronic infections or inflammatory disorders. The amyloid protein is derived from serum amyloid A-related protein. This protein is synthesized in inflammatory states and if present for long enough at a high enough level becomes deposited in various organs.

Table 11.1 The differences between myeloma and MGUS.

	Myeloma	**MGUS**
Bone marrow plasma cells	>10% on bone marrow aspirate	<10% on bone marrow aspirate
Serum paraprotein	Usually high and rising	Usually low and stable
Bence-Jones proteinuria	>50% of cases	Rare
Immune paresis	Very common	Rare
Lytic bone lesions	Common	Absent
Hypercalcaemia	Common	Absent
Anaemia	Frequent	Absent
Impaired renal function	May be present	Absent

Note: Treatment is not indicated for patients with MGUS. Randomized trials have clearly demonstrated that there is no benefit from early intervention and simple monitoring of the paraprotein with clinical review is all that is required.

2 *AL amyloid*: These proteins consist of part or whole of the immunoglobulin light chain. The classical features include macroglossia, carpal tunnel syndrome, peripheral neuropathy and purpura, but more important clinically are malabsorption, nephrotic syndrome and cardiomyopathy. Patients are found to have monoclonal light chain excretion. They may have an increased number of plasma cells in the bone marrow but do not have bone lesions.

Few effective treatment modalities exist and prognosis is therefore poor (especially in patients with cardiac infiltration). Where treatment is given it is usually derived from the protocols used for patients with myeloma.

3 *Familial forms*: This is a diverse group of diseases, often presenting as neuropathy but frequently involving other organs.

Waldenström's macroglobulinaemia (see Chapter 10, p. 110)

Waldenstrom's macroglobulinaemia (or lymphoplasmacytoid lymphoma) is also characterized by the presence of a paraprotein, although, in contrast to myeloma, in this condition it is nearly always IgM. The paraprotein is secreted by a clonal population of cells derived from the B-cell lineage, their precise identity being uncertain. Morphologically, these cells appear to be plasmacytoid lymphocytes, and they may be found in peripheral lymphoid tissue, bone marrow and, in some patients, the peripheral blood. Symptoms result both from tissue infiltration and from hyperviscosity of the blood caused by the paraprotein. Osteolytic lesions are rare. It is a relatively uncommon condition, being found at approximately 10% of the incidence of myeloma.

Heavy chain diseases

In these rare paraproteinaemias, the B lineage-derived malignant clone secretes γ, α or μ heavy chains rather than complete Ig molecules. The clinical picture is that of a lymphoma; α-chain disease is characterized by severe malabsorption due to infiltration of the small intestine by lymphoma cells.

Other lymphoproliferative disorders

A paraprotein may also be found in chronic cold haemagglutinin disease, and in some patients with malignant lymphoma or chronic lymphocytic leukaemia.

Chapter 12

Neoplastic Disorders of Myeloid Cells

Learning objectives

- To understand the presentation, natural history and diagnosis of acute myeloblastic leukaemia.
- To have an understanding of the myelodysplastic disorders.
- To be familiar with the term myeloproliferative disorder and the four main types – chronic myeloid leukaemia, polycythaemia vera, myelofibrosis and essential thrombocythaemia.
- To appreciate the expanding scientific understanding of these conditions.

Myeloid cells include granulocytic (sometimes called myeloid), erythroid and megakaryocytic cell lineages all of which are thought to arise from a single multipotent common stem cell. The earliest morphologically recognizable cell in the granulocytic lineage is called the myeloblast. The myeloblast differentiates to become a promyelocyte with the appearance of azurophilic granules. Further maturation sees the appearance of specific granules and disappearance of blast-like features. The cells at this stage are known as myelocytes, eosinophil myelocytes, basophil myelocytes and neutrophil myelocytes. The neutrophil myelocyte divides

and the progeny develop into metamyelocytes and finally mature neutrophils, as outlined on p. 11. These later stages are characterized by the involution of the nucleus as it becomes less spherical and more band-like. Monocytes are derived from promonocytes that are recognizable morphologically. The earliest erythroid cell that can be identified morphologically within the bone marrow is the pronormoblast. These large cells with dark blue cytoplasm mature and divide to become normoblasts, reticulocytes and finally mature red cells. Megakaryocytes are large multinucleated cells that derive from megakaryoblasts, which give rise to platelets by cytoplasmic shedding (Chapter 1).

A neoplastic clone can emerge from any of these stages although the more mature cells are less often involved in the neoplastic process. The malignant process may be obvious with large numbers of blast cells — *acute myeloid leukaemia (AML)*. Other disorders can be divided, with some overlap, into *myelodysplastic* and *myeloproliferative* conditions. The myelodysplastic disorders are characterized by abnormal morphology (dysplasia) with altered function; there is often an excess of blast cells the abnormalities terminating as a florid leukaemia. The myeloproliferative disorders are characterized by increased numbers of cells with relatively normal morphology and function. The myeloproliferative disorders may also transform to acute leukaemia but this is an uncommon event.

Lecture Notes: Haematology, by NC Hughes-Jones, SN Wickramsinghe, CSR Hatton © 2008 Blackwell Publishing, ISBN: 9781405180504

Table 12.1 WHO 2001 classification of AML.

Acute myeloblastic leukaemia with recurrent cytogenetic changes	AML with t(8;21); inv16 t(15;17); all mostly occurring in young patients
AML with multilineage dysplasia	Evolving from a myelodysplastic disorder; mostly occurring in older patients
AML and MDSs, therapy related	Alkylating agent related, topoisomerase II inhibitor related
AML not otherwise categorized	Morphologically classified M0–M7 as previously according to cell of origin

Notes: AML—acute myeloid leukaemia; MDSs—myelodysplastic syndromes.

Acute myeloid leukaemia

AML is a clonal disorder of myeloid progenitor cells that may occur at any age but becomes increasingly common in older people. It is the most common form of acute leukaemia in adults. The disorder leads to an infiltration of the bone marrow with immature cells leading to impaired production of neutrophils, platelets and red cells. Blast cells frequently appear in the peripheral blood and may derive from any of the lineages described above. The classification of the disorder is based on morphology, cytogenetics, immunophenotyping and clinical behaviour, reminiscent of the classification of lymphoid disorders.

Aetiology

The vast majority of cases have no identifiable aetiology though a number of cases may evolve from other clonal myeloid disorders such as the myelodysplastic disorders and the myeloproliferative conditions. Radiation and benzene exposure are also known to lead to AML. There are rare incidences where individuals have a predisposition to AML. Children affected with Down's syndrome have a 400 times higher incidence of AML (M7) compared with unaffected children. In addition there are families that have inherited mutations of critical haematopoietic transcription factors (e.g. AML-1) that may give rise to AML.

Classification

The malignant cells are thought to represent neoplastic equivalents of normal maturation stages and eight types are recognized by the well recognized FAB classification:

1 Undifferentiated blasts: M0
2 Lightly granulated blasts: M1
3 Granulated blasts often with Auer rods: M2
4 Promyelocytic leukaemia: M3
5 Myelomonocytic leukaemia: M4
6 Monocytic leukaemia: M5
7 Erythroleukaemia: M6
8 Megakaryocytic leukaemia: M7.

Previous attempts at classifying AML have been based on the morphological features described above. However, as the underlying molecular abnormalities which give rise to AML become better understood, attempts are being made to produce a more scientifically coherent classification. The WHO classification therefore attempts to classify AML by its underlying molecular abnormalities (e.g. recurrent cytogenetic changes). The complexities of this new classification, given in Table 12.1, reflect our incomplete knowledge of the molecular basis in many cases of AML.

Symptoms and signs

The clinical features reflect the consequences of *bone marrow failure*. Thus, anaemia causes pallor, tiredness and exertional dyspnoea; leucopenia leads to infection; and thrombocytopenia causes bleeding, bruising and purpura. Blast cells may infiltrate other organs such as the skin, gums (particularly in monocytic leukaemia), and there may be lymph adenopathy and splenomegaly. Massive splenomegaly is unusual in this disorder. Blast cells can invade the CNS, although this is commoner at relapse.

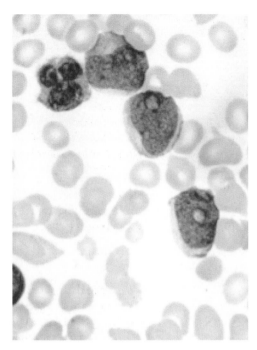

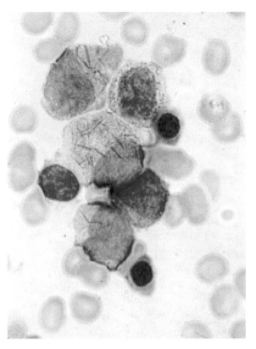

Figure 12.1 AML (FAB category M1); the three leukaemic myeloblasts are considerably larger than adjacent red cells, have finely stippled nuclear chromatin and show prominent nucleoli (MGG (May–Grünwald–Giemsa) stain).

Figure 12.2 Myeloblasts of AML showing several Auer rods (MGG stain). These are azurophilic rod-shaped cytoplasmic inclusions that are exclusively found in some of the leukaemic myeloblasts of a small proportion of patients with AML, or CML in blast-cell transformation.

Laboratory findings

Laboratory findings, like the clinical findings, reflect bone marrow failure. Anaemia results from inadequate red cell production. Thrombocytopenia is nearly always present and results both from a failure of production and increased consumption. Some cases of AML are associated with disseminated intravascular coagulation (DIC). The white cell count may be very high reflecting the high circulating blast-cell count but in about half the patients the total white cell count is low. In almost all cases the total number of normal circulating neutrophils is reduced.

The bone marrow always contains blast cells often accounting for more than 90% of the nucleated cells (Fig. 12.1).

AML must be distinguished from acute lymphoblastic leukaemia (ALL) because the treatment and management differ. The morphological features may be diagnostic but in cases where the

blast cells are not well differentiated and lack granules, the cytochemical demonstration of certain intracellular enzymes or expression of a typical antigen profile by immunophenotyping may be required. *Auer rods* are needle-shaped or rod-shaped cytoplasmic inclusions (formed by fusion of granules) within blast cells and are virtually diagnostic of AML (Fig. 12.2).

Immunophenotyping using flow cytometry is a method whereby the antigen profile of the leukaemic cells can be identified (see p. 81 and Fig. 12.3). Myeloid antigens such as CD13, CD15, CD33, the stem cell marker CD34 and stem cell factor receptor c-kit (CD117) help to identify blast cells as myeloid rather than lymphoid. The lymphoblasts in ALL will express B- or T-cell markers.

AML with recurrent genetic abnormalities

A number of characteristic cytogenetic abnormalities occur in AML. Their importance in terms of

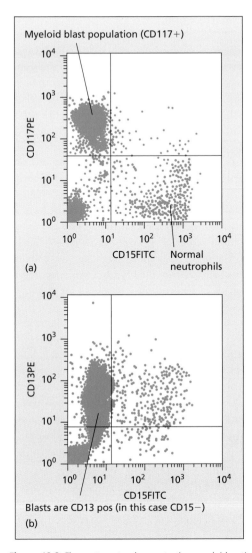

Figure 12.3 Flow cytometry demonstrating myeloid antigen expression in a case of AML. The blasts are CD117+ and CD13+.

Table 12.2 Cytogenetic abnormalities that have been found to be associated with a good prognosis in AML.

Translocation t(8;21)	Found in granulocytic variant of AML; the blast cells have obvious granules and Auer rods are frequently present
Translocation t(15;17)	Defines acute promyelocytic leukaemia (APML). The leukaemic promyelocytes are heavily granulated with prominent Auer rods. This type is associated with a severe coagulopathy
Inversion Inv(16)	Occurs in myelomonocytic leukaemia with an excess of eosinophils in the bone marrow

of mutated nucleophosmin (NPM1) is present in half of cytogenetically normal AML and is associated with a relatively good prognosis. Current research is uncovering point mutations in critical haemopoietic transcription factors (CEBPα and GATA-1). The prevalence and clinical significance of these mutations is a matter of debate.

Therapy-related AML has been recognized as a late complication of chemotherapy. In these patients there is a recurring abnormality of chromosome 5 and/or 7 (-5/del(5q) or -7/del(7q)). Patients who have received topoisomerase II inhibitors (etoposide) have a high incidence of balanced translocations involving 11q23 and 21q22. Therapy-related AML has a very poor prognosis.

Acute promyelocytic leukaemia (M3)

This variant deserves special mention not only because it has specific clinical manifestations but also because of the molecular understanding of the disorder. The malignant cells in acute promyelocytic leukaemia (APML) are promyelocytes that contain abundant granules and numerous Auer rods. Release of the promyelocytes' granules, which may occur spontaneously or at the initiation of cytotoxic therapy, is known to produce uncontrolled activation of the fibrinolytic system. The result is DIC, and potentially life-threatening bleeding.

causation is obvious but it is also now well established that certain abnormalities are associated with useful prognostic information (Table 12.2).

In addition to these 'classic' cytogenetic abnormalities, research is uncovering additional mutations of prognostic significance. Mutations of a cytokine receptor (FLT-3) are thought to impart an adverse prognosis. In some series up to 30% of cases carry such mutations. Abnormal localization

Treatment with alltrans-retinoic acid (ATRA) allows differentiation of the abnormal promyelocytes, and limits the threat of DIC. This differentiating agent alone allow some patients to reach remission, although most will subsequently relapse. The combination of ATRA with conventional chemotherapy has made APML the most curable subtype of AML.

The molecular basis of APML and the sensitivity of the disorder to ATRA are of considerable interest. The disorder is characterized by a translocation between chromosome 15 and chromosome 17. The breakpoint on chromosome 17 falls within the gene for the retinoic acid receptor (*RARα*), which is normally needed for appropriate differentiation of the cell. The breakpoint on chromosome 15 falls within the gene known as *PML*, a nuclear regulatory factor needed to control the induction of apoptosis of the cell. As a result of the translocation a new fusion gene called *RARα/PML* is produced, which encodes a novel retinoic acid receptor. Instead of differentiating in response to normal levels of retinoic acid, the cell remains at the promyelocyte stage and continues to proliferate. Pharmacological doses of retinoic acid (ATRA) can overcome this block, and allow normal differentiation to take place.

Treatment of AML

The treatment of AML can be divided into four main components: intensive chemotherapy, supportive care, differentiation agents and bone marrow transplantation (BMT).

Intensive chemotherapy

The use of anthracycline drugs together with cytosine arabinoside leads to remissions in up to 80% of younger patients. Following administration of chemotherapy there is a disappearance of circulating blast cells and a temporary worsening of the cytopenias leading to severe neutropenia and thrombocytopenia. Elderly patients have lower rates of remission and generally have a poor prognosis — patients over 70 years of age rarely survive beyond 1 year due to resistant disease or to complications of therapy.

Supportive care

Following chemotherapy there is an inevitable period of neutropenia associated with a breakdown of mucosal surfaces; patients commonly complain of a sore throat and dysphagia and may develop abdominal pain as a result of inflammation of the bowel mucosa. This is the period when the patient is susceptible to overwhelming septicaemia (neutropenic sepsis); the infection most often arises from damaged mucosal surfaces of the gut, in particular the large bowel, allowing the passage of Gram-negative organisms into the blood stream. The presence of fever or other features of infection should lead to prompt administration of intravenous antibiotics aimed at Gram-negative organisms. The intensity of the chemotherapy used to treat AML may lead to periods of neutropenia continuing for as long as 3–4 weeks. Such extended periods of neutropenia are associated with fungal infection, notably invasive *Aspergillus* and *Candida* species. Prophylactic antifungal treatment helps reduce *Candida* infection. Platelet and red cell transfusions are necessary until normal haematopoiesis is restored. Additional courses of chemotherapy will reduce the blast count still further and can lead to durable remissions in a significant number of cases.

Bone marrow transplantation (see Chapter 13)

For patients with features indicating poor risk disease or who have relapsed, BMT may be curative. Allogeneic BMT relies on using myeloablative therapy (which may involve treatment with either drugs alone or a combination of drugs and radiotherapy); it aims to destroy the patient's bone marrow and considerably reduce the number of malignant blast cells. Immunosuppression allows the HLA-matched donor bone marrow to engraft, usually in 2–3 weeks. The donor marrow can then induce a 'graft versus leukaemia effect' — an immunological effect that eradicates chemoresistant disease.

The myelodysplastic syndromes

The myelodysplastic syndromes (MDSs) are serious, relatively common disorders in which the bone marrow is populated by a clone of abnormal haemopoietic cells. These cells are dysplastic and are unable to mature normally. The maturation block tends to worsen over time leading to an accumulation of blast cells. Ultimately, the disorder may lead to bone marrow failure, either as a result of a transformation to acute leukaemia, or because of stem cell failure. The marrow blast-cell count is the single most important factor in determining prognosis, with a higher blast count conferring a poorer prognosis. The disease is most common in the elderly and is rare before the age of 50 years. MDS presents most commonly with symptoms of anaemia but infection, bruising or bleeding may also occur. MDS has been subdivided into a number of categories depending on the presence of underlying cytogenetic abnormalities and morphological features such as ring sideroblasts.

Laboratory features

Typically, there is reduction in at least two cell lines (e.g. anaemia and leucopenia, or anaemia and thrombocytopenia). The anaemia is frequently macrocytic (not due to vitamin B_{12} or folate deficiency) and the neutrophils are 'dysplastic' — they look bizarre, often with reduced granulation and abnormal nuclear maturation, including the characteristic bilobed spectacle-like nuclei (Fig. 12.4).

Blasts cells may be found in the peripheral blood. An increase in peripheral blood monocytes ($>1 \times 10^9$/L) in some cases defines these patients as having *chronic myelomonocytic leukaemia* (CMML).

The bone marrow has variable cellularity though there is always abnormal maturation easily recognized by microscopy. The blast count may vary from less than 5% in *refractory anaemia* (RA), to more than 5% blasts *in refractory anaemia with excess blasts* (RAEB). A blast-cell count greater than 20% in the bone marrow defines the condition as acute leukaemia. The presence of iron granules in the mitochondria of erythroid precursors (nucleated red cells) forming a ring of iron-positive granules around the nucleus defines the condition known as *primary acquired sideroblastic anaemia* or *refractory anaemia with ring sideroblasts* (RARS). Cytogenetic abnormalities occur in about 50% of cases.

Treatment

Treatment is usually supportive only, as this condition responds poorly to chemotherapy. Many patients are transfusion dependent. In younger patients, chemotherapy and BMT may be the treatment of choice. Trials have shown that certain growth factors such as erythropoietin and granulocyte stimulatory agents (G-CSF) can alleviate the associated cytopenias in certain subgroups

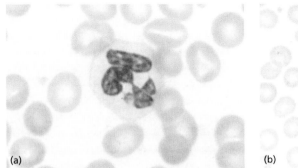

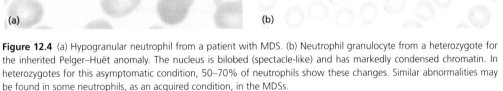

(a) (b)

Figure 12.4 (a) Hypogranular neutrophil from a patient with MDS. (b) Neutrophil granulocyte from a heterozygote for the inherited Pelger–Huët anomaly. The nucleus is bilobed (spectacle-like) and has markedly condensed chromatin. In heterozygotes for this asymptomatic condition, 50–70% of neutrophils show these changes. Similar abnormalities may be found in some neutrophils, as an acquired condition, in the MDSs.

of patients with MDS. Other subgroups of MDS have been shown to respond to the immunomodulatory agent lenalidamide though the mechanism is not understood.

Myeloproliferative disorders

The myeloproliferative disorders are a group of diseases in which there is increased proliferative activity with fairly normal maturation, unlike the MDSs. Functional abnormalities of the blood cells are usually mild but there may be an increase in the numbers of neutrophils, erythrocytes or platelets.

The myeloproliferative disorders are chronic myeloid leukaemia (CML), polycythaemia vera, myelofibrosis and essential thrombocythaemia.

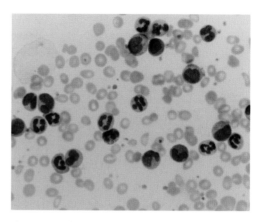

Figure 12.5 Blood film from a patient with CML showing increased number of white cells, mainly neutrophils, band cells and metamyelocytes. Note the presence of some myelocytes and basophils.

Chronic myeloid leukaemia

CML is very rare in children but increases in incidence with age. The most frequent symptoms are those of fatigue, weight loss, sweats and anorexia. The commonest signs are pallor and sometimes massive splenomegaly. Very occasionally CML may present with symptoms of hyperviscosity due to a very high white cell count. Priapism, tinnitus and stupor are among the commoner symptoms of this presentation.

Laboratory features

The peripheral blood abnormalities are characteristic. Patients are almost always anaemic and have elevated white cell counts (usually between 50 and 400×10^9/L) with excess neutrophils, myelocytes, metamyelocytes and basophils present in the peripheral blood (Fig. 12.5); blast cells are also present in small numbers (<5%). The bone marrow is very hypercellular with greatly increased white cell production.

Clinical course

The disorder runs a predictable course. In the first phase (the '*chronic phase*'), normal blood counts are achieved with therapy and the patient is generally

well. This phase may continue for many years. Inevitably the disease then transforms through an *accelerated phase* (blood counts difficult to control) into *blast crisis*. This latter phase is defined by an increasing number of blasts in the bone marrow, and in terms of its natural history, is akin to acute leukaemia. Symptomatically, patients describe weight loss, night sweats and fevers. Some patients in blast crisis may be rescued with conventional chemotherapy and enter a second chronic phase.

Philadelphia chromosome

CML is associated with a pathognomonic chromosomal rearrangement in which there is a reciprocal translocation between chromosome 22 and chromosome 9. This leads to the formation of a novel gene that is transcribed into a novel oncoprotein with tyrosine kinase activity (BCR–ABL) (Fig. 12.6(a)). This protein leads to increased cell cycling and a failure of apoptosis. The fusion chromosome 22q– (with additional material from chromosome 9) is known as the *Philadelphia chromosome*. In 1990, two experimental approaches demonstrated the ability of the *BCR–ABL* fusion gene (as the sole abnormality) to cause leukaemia. First, transgenic mice that express the *BCR–ABL* gene have been shown to develop a rapidly fatal acute leukaemia; second, when murine bone

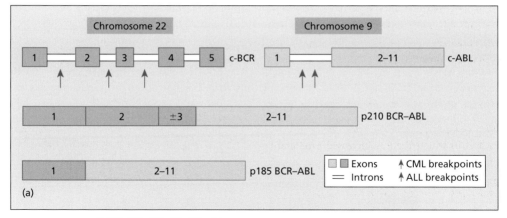

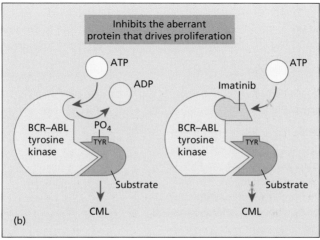

Figure 12.6 (a) Diagram to illustrate the translocation between chromosomes 22 and 9 leading to the formation of a novel oncogene *BCR–ABL*. Note a variation of the same translocation occurs in some patients with ALL. The novel oncogene produces a tyrosine kinase leading to cell proliferation. (b) Diagram showing the mechanism of action of imatinib. This drug inhibits the phosphorylation by BCR–ABL of tyrosine in protein (shown in green), and thereby interferes with its leukaemogenic effects.

marrow cells transfected with a BCR–ABL expressing retrovirus were used to repopulate the bone marrow of irradiated mice, the mice developed various myeloproliferative disorders including CML.

These observations have led to the concept that the tyrosine kinase BCR–ABL is a target for therapy. Inhibitors of the ATP-binding site on this tyrosine kinase have therefore been developed to treat CML. One such compound that finally emerged as a specific inhibitor of BCR–ABL was STI571, now known as imatinib (Glivec®), which has transformed the management of chronic phase CML (Fig. 12.6(b)). By blocking the inactive conformation of the BCR–ABL oncoprotein, imatinib allows inhibition of its oncogenetic activity and thereby treats CML at the molecular level.

Treatment

The majority of patients with CML will respond to imatinib therapy with normalization of their blood counts and reduction of their enlarged spleens. Furthermore, over 80% of patients will achieve a cytogenetic remission and may remain in remission for many years. Imatinib is relatively well tolerated and only a handful of patients are resistant. Those patients who are resistant to imatinib can be treated with second line tyrosine kinase inhibitors such as dasatinib which targets the active conformation of the tyrosine kinase. CML provides an outstanding example of the effectiveness of targeted therapy where the understanding of molecular mechanisms has enabled the development of specific drugs to block offending oncogenic proteins.

Whilst imatinib will provide control of CML in many cases, it cannot cure the disease. Allogeneic BMT is the only known curative therapy for this disorder and is most successfully carried out in chronic phase. This procedure is not available to patients over the age of 45–50 years and relies on being able to identify a tissue-matched donor, either a sibling or an unrelated matched donor. The majority of patients with CML will not be found to have a suitable matched donor or will be too old for allogeneic BMT.

Polycythaemia vera

This chronic clonal disorder is characterized by excessive proliferation of a multipotent haemopoietic stem cell, resulting in an increased number of red cells, often accompanied by an increase in white cell and platelet counts. The primary clinical manifestation is markedly elevated haemoglobin and haematocrit. The clonal nature of the abnormal cells has been known for some time but now a defining mutation in the erythropoietin signaling pathway (JAK2) has been identified. This mutation has been found in over 90% of cases of polycythaemia vera and JAK2 mutational analysis has become an important diagnostic test in this disorder.

Clinical features

Polycythaemia vera has an insidious onset, usually presenting late in life (rarely before 40 years). The main presenting symptoms relate to the considerable rise in red cell count and resulting increase in blood viscosity and include headache, dizziness and, sometimes, stroke. Pruritus, particularly after hot baths is a characteristic symptom. There is a marked tendency for patients to develop thrombosis though there may also be an increased likelihood of bleeding. Mesenteric, portal or splenic vein thrombosis should alert the clinician to the possibility of polycythaemia vera. The principal signs are those of plethora (florid dusky red colour of the face), splenomegaly and hepatomegaly. Erythromelalgia (increased skin temperature, burning sensation and redness) may occur in the extremities.

Laboratory findings and natural history

The red cell count and haemoglobin concentration are increased; haemoglobin values of 18–24 g/dL are common and the packed cell volume (PCV) is usually over 0.48 in females and 0.51 in males; the red cell mass (measured using ^{51}Cr-labelled red cells) is increased. An increase in the white cell count occurs in the majority of patients and about 50% of patients have an elevated platelet count.

Most patients with polycythaemia vera will remain well in the so-called 'plethoric' phase, providing the haematocrit is controlled by venesection. Furthermore, many patients can expect to have a normal life expectancy. Eventually the marrow may become increasingly fibrotic (myelofibrosis) leading to a fall in the haematocrit, increasing splenomegaly and often a requirement for blood transfusion in the later stages.

There are various cytogenetic abnormalities in the bone marrow cells of some cases but no consistent abnormality has been detected.

Differential diagnosis

Secondary polycythaemia is the main differential diagnosis for polycythaemia vera. Longstanding hypoxia caused by cardiopulmonary disease or living at high altitudes will lead to an increased red cell mass and therefore a high haemoglobin and haematocrit (see Chapter 2). However, the elevated haematocrit and haemoglobin are usually the only haematological abnormality; where leucocytosis, thrombocytosis and splenomegaly are also found polycythaemia vera is more likely. Some patients may have a high haematocrit as a result of a reduction in the plasma volume (e.g. due to diuretics). So-called *apparent polycythaemia* can be differentiated from polycythaemia vera and secondary polycythaemia by measurement of the red cell mass and the plasma volume. The JAK2 mutation which characterizes nearly all cases of polycythaemia vera is seldom present in secondary or apparent polycythaemia.

Treatment

The mainstay of treatment is venesection, aiming to lower the haematocrit below 0.50, and preferably below 0.45, thus preventing thrombotic episodes. In the early stages this may have to be performed at least twice weekly. Low-dose aspirin is also frequently used to minimize the risk of stroke. Patients with significant leucocytosis or thrombocytosis can be treated with cytoreductive therapy using oral chemotherapy agents such as hydroxycarbamide or busulphan. A single injection of radioactive phosphorus (^{32}P) can be very effective in controlling the red cell counts, but the significant risk of inducing secondary leukaemia has made this agent unpopular.

Primary myelofibrosis

This is a clonal disorder of the haematopoietic stem cell which typically occurs after the age of 50 years. It is characterized by splenomegaly (which may be massive), immature circulating cells in the blood (nucleated red cells and myelocytes), distorted red cells (so-called teardrop cells). These findings are due to the defining feature of myelofibrosis, bone marrow fibrosis. The marrow fibrosis is reactive and non-clonal and is thought to be secondary to the abnormal haemopoiesis. At the molecular level approximately 50% of patients with primary myelofibrosis harbor the JAK2 mutation that has been identified in patients with primary polycythaemia. In other patients, mutations affecting the thrombopoietin receptor have been described. Many patients with an identical phenotype and with clonal haematopoiesis do not have either of these mutations and it is therefore impossible to know the full relevance of these findings to date.

The disorder may transform to acute leukaemia. Although the principal site of extramedullary haemopoiesis is the spleen or liver, other sites such as the lymph nodes, adrenal or dura may be involved.

Clinical features

This disorder usually presents in patients over the age of 50 years but can occasionally occur in children. Patients may present with constitutional symptoms such as weight loss, night sweats or fever. Other presenting symptoms include 'splenic' pain, or symptoms due to anaemia such as fatigue, shortness of breath and palpitations. Occasional patients may present with gout as a consequence of hyperuricaemia resulting from the high cell turnover. Presenting signs include hepatomegaly, splenomegaly (nearly all cases) and pallor.

Laboratory findings

Normochromic normocytic anaemia is found in most patients with myelofibrosis. Leucocytosis and thrombocytosis are common findings although the total white cell count is not usually as high as that found in CML and is rarely over 40×10^9/L. Inspection of the blood film is often diagnostic. The blood film typically shows the presence of normoblasts and myelocytes (i.e. a leucoerythroblastic picture, with the presence of teardrop poikilocytes (Fig. 12.7)). Bone marrow

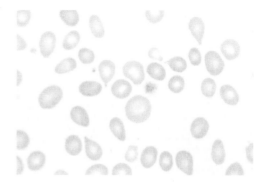

Figure 12.7 Blood film of a patient with idiopathic myelofibrosis showing several teardrop-shaped poikilocytes and an abnormally large platelet (MGG stain).

131

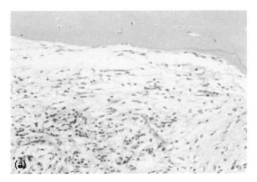 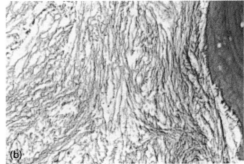

Figure 12.8 (a) Trephine biopsy of the bone marrow of a patient with idiopathic myelofibrosis showing fibroblasts and collagen fibrosis (haematoxylin and eosin). (b) Section of the same trephine biopsy showing increased reticulin fibres (silver impregnation of reticulin).

aspiration is often unsuccessful because of the fibrosis, resulting in a dry tap. The bone marrow biopsy shows myeloproliferation with granulocytic and megakaryocytic hyperplasia together with fibrosis, which may be dense (Fig. 12.8).

Treatment

Many patients need no specific treatment but patients with a more proliferative marrow may require cytoreductive treatment with a gentle chemotherapy drug such as oral daily hydroxycarbamide. Monitoring of the patient's blood count is necessary in all cases. Most patients will become transfusion dependent and, as in the case of any patient requiring regular transfusion, iron loading of tissues may occur. Massive splenic enlargement can give rise to pain which may necessitate splenectomy. Removal of the spleen may reduce transfusion requirements. The median survival of patients with myelofibrosis is in the order of 5 years from the time of diagnosis but some patients may survive for many years. The only curative therapy for primary myelofibrosis is allogeneic stem cell transplantation. A number of series have demonstrated the feasibility of reduced intensity conditioned allografting in high-risk patients. Clearly many patients with this disorder will either be too old for stem cell transplant or will have low-risk indolent disease. Causes of death in patients with primary myelofibrosis include infection, haemorrhage or transformation to acute leukaemia.

Table 12.3 Causes of thrombocytosis.

Reactive
- Haemorrhage, haemolysis, trauma, surgery, postpartum, recovery from thrombocytopenia
- Acute and chronic infections
- Chronic inflammatory disease (e.g. ulcerative colitis, rheumatoid arthritis)
- Malignant disease (e.g. carcinoma, Hodgkin's disease)
- Splenectomy and splenic atrophy
- Iron deficiency anaemia

Chronic myeloproliferative disorders
- Essential thrombocythaemia, polycythaemia vera, chronic myeloid leukaemia, idiopathic myelofibrosis

Essential thrombocythaemia

This is a clonal myeloproliferative disorder that chiefly involves the megakaryocyte cell line. The disorder is classically associated with a marked rise in the platelet count; the haemoglobin concentration, and the white cell count usually being unaffected. Many patients are diagnosed by the incidental finding of thrombocytosis during the course of a routine blood count. The difficulty arises in differentiating this condition from reactive causes of thrombocytosis (Table 12.3) as there is no specific diagnostic test for essential thrombocythaemia (Table 12.4). Approximately 50% of patients with ET have the common JAK2 mutation that has been identified in patients

Table 12.4 Diagnostic criteria for essential thrombocythaemia.

> - Platelet count >600 × 10^9/L (sustained)
> - ET bone marrow changes — proliferation of megakaryocytes
> Exclusion of
>   Polycythaemia vera
>   Primary myelofibrosis
>   CML
>   MDS
> - No known cause for reactive thrombocytosis

with primary polycythaemia and primary myelofibrosis. It is not yet clear how this single mutation can give rise to these three distinct disease entities.

Clinical features

This is a disorder that affects older patients, usually presenting with thrombotic or bleeding complications. Many patients are asymptomatic at presentation. Older patients seem to be at greater risk of thrombosis, particularly arterial. The main thrombotic complications are:

1 Erythromelalgia and digital ischaemia. Erythromelalgia is characterized by intense burning and pain in the extremities. The pain is increased by exercise, warmth or dependency. The extremities are warm with mottled erythema. Digital ischaemia mainly affects the toes. Such vascular insufficiency sometimes leads to gangrene and loss of function.
2 Stroke.
3 Recurrent abortions and fetal growth retardation.
4 Hepatic and portal vein thrombosis. The myeloproliferative disorders are the most common causes of hepatic vein thrombosis (Budd–Chiari syndrome).

Laboratory findings

A raised platelet count, often over 1000 × 10^9/L, is characteristic of the disorder. The bone marrow shows increased cellularity and plentiful megakaryocytes but the changes are not specific to the disorder and may occur in reactive states. The diagnosis remains one of exclusion. Certain criteria must be satisfied before the diagnosis can be entertained and these are listed in Table 12.4.

Treatment

Treatment of essential thrombocythaemia is ill-defined. There may not be any necessity to treat a young asymptomatic patient and most authorities suggest a risk-based approach. Patients over the age of 60 years or with a platelet count greater than 1000 × 10^9/L should be considered for active treatment. The following agents have been used:

1 Simple oral chemotherapy with hydroxycarbamide or busulphan for elderly patients.
2 α-interferon reduces platelet counts but may cause unacceptable side effects such as fatigue, fever, pyrexia and depression. It is the treatment of choice in women of childbearing age due its relative safety in pregnancy.
3 Anagrelide: This agent inhibits megakaryocyte maturation and does not affect the white cell count. It is the preferred treatment in some centres, but can cause vasodilatation, cardiac dysrhythmias and fluid retention.

Antiplatelet drugs such as aspirin can be highly effective in patients at risk of thrombotic episodes. They may be associated with haemorrhage and should not be used in patients with a bleeding tendency.

The survival of patients with essential thrombocythaemia is similar to that of an age-matched population.

Chapter 13

Bone Marrow Transplantation

Learning objectives

- To understand the use of stem cell infusion following high dose or myeloablative chemotherapy.
- To understand the concept of the graft versus leukaemia/lymphoma effect.
- To understand the nature of graft versus host disease.

The idea of rescuing patients by infusing bone marrow after myeloablative chemotherapy or radiotherapy is not a new concept. Animal experiments carried out in the 1950s demonstrated that intravenous infusion of marrow cells could protect against lethal irradiation. Subsequently, successful engraftment was demonstrated in humans.

Bone marrow transplantation may be autologous or allogeneic. In autologous transplantation, the patient's own stem cells are collected following standard chemotherapy treatment. Doses of cytotoxic treatment which ablate the bone marrow are then administered, followed by reinfusion of the collected stem cells. These stem cells repopulate the bone marrow and allow recovery from otherwise supra-lethal doses of chemotherapy or radiotherapy (Table 13.1).

The understanding of the human leucocyte antigen system (HLA) meant that tissue matching between donor and patient was possible and successful bone marrow transplants (BMTs) using

Lecture Notes: Haematology, by NC Hughes-Jones, SN Wickramsinghe, CSR Hatton © 2008 Blackwell Publishing, ISBN: 9781405180504

matched donors (*allogeneic BMT*) followed in increasing numbers (Fig. 13.1). Allogeneic transplantation was initially assumed to be beneficial because it allowed the administration of doses of cytotoxic treatments which would otherwise have been lethal, totally ablating the native bone marrow, as in autologous transplantation. However, it has since emerged that a critical component of the effectiveness of allogeneic transplantation is the immunologically mediated 'graft-versus-leukaemia' (GVL) effect, whereby T cells infused as part of the BMT exert a direct anti-tumour effect. Where there is no immunological difference of donor and recipient, as in identical twin-sibling transplants, there is a higher relapse rate than when a non-twin-sibling matched donor is used; this highlights the importance of the GVL effect in the success of allogeneic transplantation. Indeed,

Table 13.1 Diseases for which allogeneic and autologous BMT may be considered.

Indications for BMT	Allogeneic BMT	Autologous BMT
Malignant		
Acute leukaemia	+	(+)
Chronic myeloid leukaemia	+	−
Lymphoma (relapsed)	(+)	+
Myeloma	+	+
Non-malignant		
Aplastic anaemia	+	−
Thalassaemia	+	−
Sickle-cell anaemia	+	−

Loan Receipt
Liverpool John Moores University
Learning and Information Services

Borrower ID: 21111120796123

Loan Date: 30/01/2009

Loan Time: 5:03 pm

Lecture notes.
31111012601421

Due Date: 06/02/2009 23:59

Please keep your receipt
in case of dispute

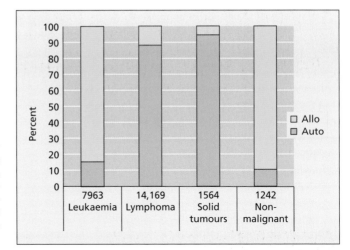

Figure 13.1 The graph shows the number and percentage of allogeneic and autologous stem cell transplants reported in Europe in 2006. The majority of allogeneic stem cell transplants are performed for AML whilst the majority of autologous transplants are performed for lymphoma.

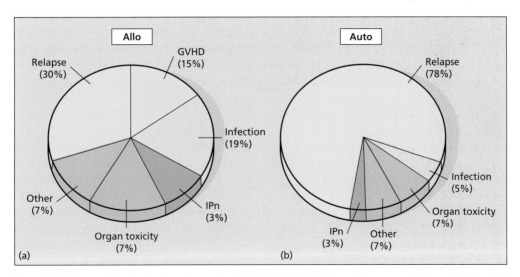

Figure 13.2 Causes of death after transplants done in 1996–2000. GVHD – graft versus host disease. IPn interstitial pneumonitis.

there is increasing reliance of the GVL effect in allogeneic transplantation as reduced-intensity conditioning (RIC) regimens become more widely used, with lower doses of cytotoxic treatment.

Allogeneic bone marrow transplantation

The necessary elements for a successful allogeneic BMT include:

1 A source of HLA-matched stem cells. Stem cells can be collected from an HLA-matched sibling,

a matched unrelated donor or in some cases matched umbilical cord blood. The chance of any sibling being a match is one in four whereas the chance of a volunteer being a match is closer to one in 100,000. Most developed countries have registers of donors against which a patient's HLA type can be matched (Fig. 13.2).

2 Immunosuppression (chemotherapy and radiotherapy) prior to marrow infusion to allow engraftment.

3 Continuing immunosuppression after infusion to prevent graft-versus-host disease (GVHD).

135

The process of allogeneic bone marrow transplantation involves:

1 *High-dose chemotherapy either with or without total body radiotherapy*: This is used to eradicate the neoplastic cells and to allow engraftment of the donor marrow.
2 *Infusion of bone marrow or peripheral blood stem cells*: These are collected directly from the bone marrow of the donor, or by leukapheresis of a donor who has been primed by growth factors such as granulocyte or granulocyte macrophage colony-stimulating factor (G-CSF, GM-CSF).
3 *Supportive care*: Following high-dose therapy there is inevitably a period of profound marrow suppression which typically lasts 2–3 weeks until the newly infused marrow engrafts. Red cells, platelets and antibiotics are essential to supportive care. Severe mucositis and gastroenteritis often develop and, consequently, many patients require parenteral nutrition during this time.
4 *Prevention of GVHD*: A number of immunosuppressive drugs are used to control the immune component (mainly T cells) of the donor-derived engrafted marrow. Ciclosporin is the mainstay of this treatment, but other drugs such as methotrexate and prednisolone are frequently used.

Complications of allogeneic BMT

The principal complication of allogeneic BMT is infection. The severe neutropenia that follows high-dose chemotherapy is frequently complicated by Gram-negative infection. Fungal (*Aspergillus* and *Candida* species) and viral (herpes viruses) infections are also found after allogeneic BMT. The use of steroids to control GVHD further increases the risk of fungal infection.

Cytomegalovirus

Cytomegalovirus (CMV) is a cause of morbidity and mortality in BMT patients. Patients may acquire active CMV infection due to the use of seropositive marrow donors, seropositive blood products or the reactivation of latent CMV infection in seropositive patients.

Infection and organ damage is related to viral load, which can be detected in the blood by the polymerase chain reaction (PCR). Interstitial pneumonitis is a serious complication of CMV infection but other organs may be affected, notably, the gastrointestinal tract. The use of CMV seronegative blood products in patients who are not already infected helps to reduce the chance of infection. Prophylactic aciclovir and the use of ganciclovir for treatment have reduced the morbidity and mortality from CMV.

Graft-versus-host disease

GVHD results from the reaction of donor T cells against the recipient's tissues; the disorder may be acute or chronic. Prophylactic ciclosporin, a T-cell inhibitor, considerably reduces the incidence and severity of GVHD and is given continuously throughout the immediate post-transplant period. Other drugs such as methotrexate and mycophenolate may be used as alternatives, or in addition to ciclosporin, to prevent GVHD.

Acute GVHD

This may occur during the first 100 days after BMT and chiefly affects the skin, gastrointestinal tract and liver. Skin involvement varies from a mild maculopapular rash to severe desquamation. Gastrointestinal involvement may involve the upper or lower tract. Symptoms include nausea, vomiting or severe watery diarrhoea. Biopsy is usually required to confirm the diagnosis.

T-cell depletion of the donor marrow reduces the risk of GVHD, and some centres routinely deplete donor marrow this way. T-cell depletion is, however, associated with a higher risk of relapse due to a reduction in the graft-versus-leukaemia effect (GVL; see below). Once established, acute GVHD is a serious disorder with a high mortality. Treatment with high-dose steroids can help but many patients with severe GVHD die of infection.

Chronic GVHD

Chronic GVHD is a serious complication of BMT occurring after 100 days in approximately 30–40% of patients. The main manifestations are those of dry eyes, skin changes, chronic liver disease, weight loss and increased risk of infection. The prognosis is poor.

Graft-versus-leukaemia/lymphoma effect

In addition to producing GVHD, the lymphocytes from the graft are also thought to exert an immune effect against the recipient's tumour cells. This is the graft-versus-leukaemia/lymphoma effect (GVL). Patients receiving a BMT for chronic myeloid leukaemia (CML) often have molecular evidence of persistent leukaemia (the presence of the Philadelphia chromosome) in the immediate post-transplant period but this later disappears, but T-cell depletion of the donor marrow is associated with a higher risk of relapse. This implies that the T cells infused with the donor stem cells are active in eradicating the underlying disease over a period of time. In the event of relapse, the infusion of lymphocytes from the original graft donor (donor lymphocyte infusion, or DLI) has been shown to have a powerful antitumour effect and may induce a further remission, at the cost of increased GVHD.

Whilst the phenomena of GVHD and GVL appear to be intimately related, the exact nature of the underlying molecular targets remains unknown. It may be that minor histocompatibility antigens are important, but evidence suggests that the explanation is more complex than this. GVHD and GVL are not necessarily produced by the same mechanisms: it is one of the key aims of research in this field to try to separate them, to harness the benefits of GVL, while avoiding the severe morbidity of GVHD. The understanding of the process of GVL should provide a powerful tool to eradicate malignant disease.

Mini-allograft or RIC transplant

Reduced intensity conditioning (RIC) allogeneic transplant relies almost entirely on engrafted donor immune cells to eradicate disease — graft-versus-leukaemia/lymphoma effect (GVL) (see above). The technique is not dependent on high-dose chemotherapy or total body irradiation to ablate malignant cells, but rather, uses lower doses of 'conditioning' therapy sufficient to allow the tissue-compatible donor stem cells to engraft. The patient is then given ciclosporin or an equivalent T-cell suppressant drug to limit the development of GVHD following donor cell engraftment. There is a balance to be struck between the benefits of GVL and the harmful effects of GVHD.

The lower dose of chemotherapy or radiotherapy reduces the toxicity and therefore the mortality of the procedure. The mini-allogeneic transplant or RIC transplant has particular relevance to an older age group since full allogeneic transplantation is limited to patients under 45–50 years of age, whereas the RIC transplant may be tolerated by patients up to the age of 65 years of age.

Extremely encouraging results for RIC allografting are emerging for low-grade lymphoproliferative and myeloproliferative disorders and trials are underway to investigate whether the immune response will be capable of controlling and destroying more aggressive disorders such as acute leukaemia.

Although more readily tolerated than full allografting, the mortality of this procedure is still in the order of between 10% and 20% in most of the reported series; the morbidity and mortality of GVHD remains a significant problem.

Autologous bone marrow transplantation (high-dose therapy)

In autologous BMT, the patient's own marrow stem cells are used to reconstitute the bone marrow after intensive chemotherapy with or without radiotherapy. There is therefore no requirement for tissue matching and the risk of GVHD is eliminated.

Chemotherapy or radiotherapy acts by killing a fraction of the tumour. Dose is, however, limited by the myeloablative effects of very high-dose treatment. This can be overcome by collecting stem cells before high-dose therapy and infusing the stem cells into the patient after intensive conditioning therapy.

There are four phases of high-dose therapy:

1 Marrow harvest/peripheral blood stem cell harvest (Fig. 13.3).

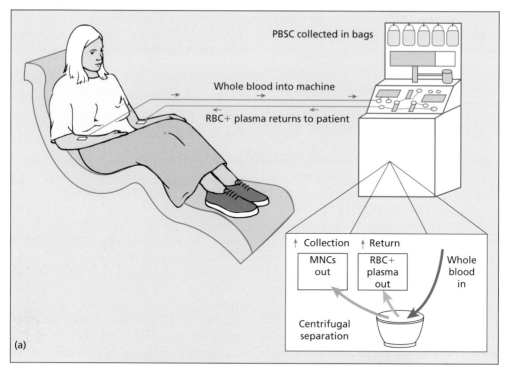

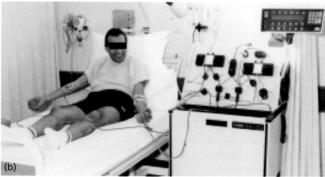

Figure 13.3 Diagram showing the collection of peripheral blood stem cells using a COBE spectra apheresis machine. *Notes*: MNC — mononuclear cells; PBSC — peripheral blood stem cells; RBC — red blood cell.

2 Conditioning therapy.

3 Reinfusion of the stem cells.

4 Supportive therapy.

Stem cells can either be collected directly by marrow puncture under general anaesthesia or by apheresis. In both cases patients need to be primed with chemotherapy and granulocyte-stimulating factor (G-CSF).

A serious disadvantage of autologous BMT is the potential for reinfusing malignant cells. Various purging strategies have been tried in an effort to reduce this risk but none has so far been shown to affect outcome positively.

Supportive therapy is very similar to the care given after any intensive chemotherapy. Blood products — red cells and platelet concentrates — together with antibiotics and nutritional support

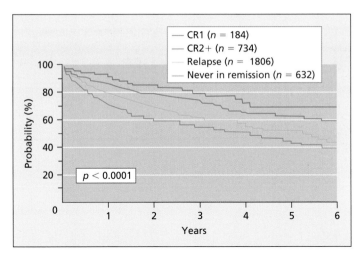

Figure 13.4 The probability of survival after autotransplants for Hodgkin Lymphoma (1994–1999). *Note*: CR — complete remission.

are the fundamentals of therapy at this stage. Most patients will engraft after 2–3 weeks, and some centres use G-CSF or GM-CSF to limit the duration of neutropenia.

The principal indications for this type of procedure include relapsed Hodgkin lymphoma (Fig. 13.4) and non-Hodgkin lymphoma and myeloma in younger patients.

Chapter 14

Aplastic Anaemia and Pure Red Cell Aplasia

Learning objectives

- To know the aetiology of acquired aplastic anaemia, including the drugs that have been most commonly reported to cause this syndrome.
- To know the clinical and laboratory features, the natural history and the principles of treatment of acquired aplastic anaemia.
- To understand the difference between aplastic anaemia and pure red cell aplasia.

Aplastic anaemia

Aplastic anaemia is a disorder characterized by pancytopenia (i.e. a reduction in the number of red cells, neutrophils and platelets in the peripheral blood), a marked decrease in the amount of haemopoietic tissue in the bone marrow (i.e. marrow aplasia or hypoplasia) and the absence of evidence of involvement of the marrow by diseases such as leukaemia, myeloma or carcinoma. The causes of aplastic anaemia are summarized in Table 14.1.

Acquired aplastic anaemia

This is an uncommon disease, the prevalence in Europe being between one and three per 100,000

people. It affects all ages with two peaks, one in adolescents and young adults and the other in people over the age of 60 years.

Aetiology

In about half the cases, no aetiological factors can be identified; such cases are described as having idiopathic acquired aplastic anaemia. In the others, the aplasia is associated with exposure to certain drugs or chemicals, ionizing radiation or certain viruses.

Most cases of secondary aplastic anaemia result from an idiosyncratic reaction to the use of antirheumatic drugs (e.g. phenylbutazone, indomethacin, ibuprofen or sodium aurothiomalate),

Table 14.1 Causes of aplastic anaemia.

Congenital
Fanconi anaemia
Acquired
Idiopathic
Drugs and chemicals
Dose-dependent: Cytotoxic drugs, benzene
Idiosyncratic: Chloramphenicol, non-steroidal anti-inflammatory drugs
Radiation
Viruses: Hepatitis non-A, non-B, non-C, Epstein–Barr virus
Paroxysmal nocturnal haemoglobinuria

Lecture Notes: Haematology, by NC Hughes-Jones, SN Wickramsinghe, CSR Hatton © 2008 Blackwell Publishing, ISBN: 9781405180504

chloramphenicol, trimethoprim-sulphamethoxazole (cotrimoxazole) or organic arsenicals. Many other drugs have been less commonly implicated and these include anticonvulsants (phenytoin, carbamazepine), antidiabetic drugs (chlorpropamide, tolbutamide), antithyroid drugs (carbimazole, propylthiouracil), mepacrine and chlorpromazine. Some drugs regularly cause aplastic anaemia if given in sufficiently large doses: these include alkylating agents (e.g. busulphan, melphalan and cyclophosphamide), antipurines, antipyrimidines and antifolates. Benzene is the only industrial chemical that often produces aplastic anaemia if inhaled in sufficient dose; kerosene, carbon tetrachloride and certain insecticides, such as DDT and chlordane, can also cause aplasia of the marrow.

Aplastic anaemia may develop after a single massive dose of whole-body irradiation (e.g. during atomic bomb explosions or radiation accidents). It was also seen in the past following repeated radiotherapy to the spine in patients with ankylosing spondylitis.

Severe aplastic anaemia, usually with a poor prognosis, may rarely develop in children and young adults about 10 weeks after an episode of acute non-A, non-B and non-C hepatitis. Marrow aplasia is also a rare complication of Epstein–Barr virus infection.

The T-lymphocytes of some patients with acquired aplastic anaemia inhibit the *in vitro* growth of haemopoietic colonies from autologous and allogeneic bone marrow. This finding, together with the response of about 50% of patients to antilymphocyte globulin, indicates that autoimmune mechanisms are involved in at least the persistence of the aplasia, if not its initiation, in a number of cases.

Pathophysiology

The pancytopenia and marrow aplasia appear to be the consequence of damage to the multipotent haemopoietic stem cells, which impairs their self-renewal (p. 8) and causes stem cell depletion. This damage may be caused by some drugs or viruses or by cell-mediated immunological mechanisms. The possibility that stromal (microenvironmental)

cell damage may be the primary defect has also been considered, but this is unlikely to be true in most cases because of the success of stem cell transplantation.

Clinical features

Both idiopathic and secondary aplastic anaemia occur at all ages. The onset is often insidious but may be acute. Symptoms include:

1 Lassitude, weakness and shortness of breath due to anaemia.
2 Haemorrhagic manifestations resulting from the thrombocytopenia.
3 Fever and recurrent infections as a consequence of neutropenia.

Haemorrhagic manifestations include epistaxis, bleeding from the gums, menorrhagia, bleeding into the gastrointestinal and urinary tracts, and ecchymoses and petechiae. The severity of the symptoms is variable and depends on the severity of the cytopenias. In patients with severe neutropenia and thrombocytopenia, fulminating infections (e.g. pneumonia) and cerebral haemorrhage are common causes of death. In secondary aplastic anaemia, symptoms may appear several weeks or months, or occasionally, 1 or more years after discontinuation of exposure to the causative drug or chemical. Splenomegaly is rare in aplastic anaemia, and if the spleen is palpable alternative diagnoses should be explored.

Haematological findings

There is a normochromic or macrocytic anaemia, associated with a low absolute reticulocyte count. The platelet count is often below $100 \times 10^9/L$, and may be very low. A neutropenia and monocytopenia are usually found at some stage of the disease. Some patients also have a reduced absolute lymphocyte count. There is a marked increase in serum and urinary erythropoietin levels.

Markedly hypocellular marrow fragments are usually found in marrow smears, most of the volume of the marrow fragments being made up

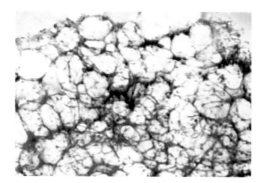

Figure 14.1 Markedly hypocellular marrow fragment from a case of aplastic anaemia. There are only a few residual haemopoietic cells, most of the fragments consisting of fat cells.

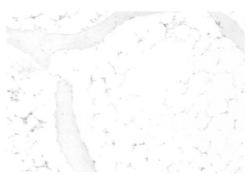

Figure 14.2 Section of a trephine biopsy of the bone marrow from a patient with aplastic anaemia showing marked hypocellularity (haemotoxylin and eosin).

of fat cells (Fig. 14.1). Haemopoietic cells of all types, including megakaryocytes, are decreased or absent, and in severe aplastic anaemia the majority of the cells seen are plasma cells, lymphocytes and macrophages. Residual erythropoietic cells are morphologically abnormal. Although the marrow is generally hypocellular, it contains some foci of normal or even increased cellularity. Thus, even in patients with severe aplastic anaemia, marrow aspiration may occasionally yield normocellular or hypercellular fragments. In order to obtain a reliable estimate of marrow cellularity, it is essential to examine histological sections of a trephine biopsy of the iliac crest (Fig. 14.2). This not only provides a larger volume of marrow for study than a single marrow aspirate but also permits the detection of foci of leukaemia cells, myeloma cells or carcinoma cells, if present.

Some patients with acquired aplastic anaemia develop the red cell defect seen in paroxysmal nocturnal haemoglobinuria (p. 46), without or with haemoglobinuria. Occasionally patients develop a terminal acute leukaemia.

Diagnosis

Other causes of pancytopenia (particularly leukaemia) should be considered and excluded before a diagnosis of aplastic anaemia is made. The causes of pancytopenia are summarized in Table 14.2.

Table 14.2 Causes of pancytopenia.

Mainly due to a failure of production of cells
Bone marrow infiltration: leukaemia, myeloma, carcinoma, myelofibrosis, lipid storage disorders, marble bone disease
Severe vitamin B_{12} or folate deficiency
Myelodysplastic syndromes
HIV infection
Aplastic or hypoplastic anaemia
Mainly due to an increased peripheral destruction of cells
Splenomegaly
Overwhelming infection
Systemic lupus erythematosus (SLE)
Paroxysmal nocturnal haemoglobinuria*

Note: * In some cases, there is also impaired production of cells due to hypoplasia of the marrow.

Prognosis

Patients with both idiopathic and secondary acquired aplastic anaemia show a highly variable clinical course. About 15% of patients have a severe illness from the outset and die within 3 months of diagnosis. Overall, as many as 50% of cases die within 15 months of diagnosis and 70% within 5 years. Only about 10% make a complete haematological recovery. If a patient survives for longer than 18 months, there is a reasonable chance of prolonged survival and complete recovery. Poor prognostic features include a platelet count less than $20 \times 10^9/L$, a neutrophil count below $0.2 \times 10^9/L$, a reticulocyte count under $10 \times 10^9/L$ and marked hypocellularity of the marrow.

Treatment

If a causative drug or chemical is identified, exposure to this agent should be immediately stopped. Supportive therapy including red cell transfusions and antibiotics should be administered when necessary; the extent of supportive therapy required depends on the degree of cytopenia. Platelet transfusions are only indicated if haemorrhage becomes a serious problem, as repeated platelet transfusions lead to alloimmunization and a reduction of the efficacy of subsequent platelet transfusions. If marrow transplantation is planned, the administration of blood products should be limited to the bare minimum, since multiple transfusions have an adverse effect on the outcome of transplantation.

Bone marrow transplantation is indicated at diagnosis for patients under 40 years with severe aplastic anaemia (i.e. showing the poor prognostic features mentioned above), particularly if an HLA-compatible sibling donor is available. Long-term survival is seen in 60–80% of cases; graft rejection is more of a problem in aplastic anaemia than in other conditions. Patients who are not transplanted may benefit from treatment with antithymocyte globulin, cyclosporin A, methylprednisolone, androgens or the anabolic steroid oxymetholone (which causes less virilization of females than androgens). Combined immunosuppressive regimens have been shown to be more effective than single-agent therapy. The addition of granulocyte colony-stimulating factor (G-CSF) has also produced encouraging results. The overall survival for patients with severe aplastic anaemia has improved considerably and is now greater than 70% at 5 years.

Pure red cell aplasia

Rarely, aplasia or severe hypoplasia affects only the erythropoietic cells. Patients with this abnormality have anaemia and reticulocytopenia together with normal white cell and platelet counts.

Fanconi anaemia

The features of this rare disorder are:

1 Inheritance as an autosomal recessive character. At least 13 different disease genes identified.
2 Onset of pancytopenia between the ages of 5 and 10 years.
3 Frequent association with other congenital abnormalities (e.g. skin pigmentation, short stature, microcephaly, skeletal defects, genital hypoplasia and renal abnormalities).
4 Various chromosomal abnormalities (breaks, rearrangements, exchanges and endoreduplications) in cultured lymphocytes and skin fibroblasts.
5 Increased number of chromosome breaks per cell after culture with alkylating agents.
6 Increased incidence of acute leukaemia and solid tumours.

There is usually some response to treatment with androgens and corticosteroids. Allogeneic bone marrow transplantation may cure the aplastic anaemia but does not prevent the appearance of solid tumours.

Table 14.3 Causes of pure red cell aplasia.

Congenital
Diamond–Blackfan syndrome (congenital erythroblastopenia or erythrogenesis imperfecta)
Acquired
Idiopathic
Viral infections: Parvovirus B19 (p. 28), Epstein–Barr virus, hepatitis
Drugs and chemicals: Phenytoin sodium, azathioprine, erythropoietin, benzene
Thymic tumours
Lymphoid malignancies: Chronic lymphocytic leukaemia, lymphoma
Other malignant diseases: Carcinoma of the bronchus, breast, stomach and thyroid
Autoimmune disorders: SLE, rheumatoid arthritis

The causes of pure red cell aplasia are listed in Table 14.3. In the rare congenital form — Diamond Blackfan anaemia — anaemia usually develops in infancy and is associated with various congenital malformations including craniofacial abnormalities and abnormalities of the thumb and upper limbs. About a quarter of cases have a mutation in the ribosome protein S19 gene.

Acquired pure red cell aplasia may present as an acute self-limiting condition (e.g. when it follows a parvovirus B19 infection) or as a chronic disorder. The reticulocytopenia that follows parvovirus B19 infection in normal individuals does not significantly lower the haemoglobin level because red cells survive for such a long time. In patients with haemolytic anaemia when red cell survival is reduced (e.g. sickle-cell anaemia), parvovirus infection leads to severe anaemia which may be life threatening. Patients with this complication present with severe pallor, white sclera (normally yellow in chronic haemolysis) and other symptoms of severe anaemia.

Immunological mechanisms, both cellular and humoral, may underlie the aplasia in some patients with chronic pure red cell aplasia (e.g. those with thymoma, chronic lymphocytic leukaemia or autoimmune disorders). A small number of patients with renal failure who have been given subcutaneous recombinant human erythropoietin have developed red cell aplasia. The mechanism is unknown but is likely to be immune mediated.

Some patients with chronic pure red cell aplasia respond to immunosuppressive drugs such as corticosteroids, azathioprine, cyclophosphamide, cyclosporin A or antithymocyte globulin. Patients with persistent parvovirus infection respond to intravenous injections of immunoglobulin.

> The parvovirus B19 enters erythroid progenitor cells (by binding to the P blood group antigen), replicates within these cells and damages them. In most patients the infection and erythroblastopenia are transient but in patients with certain congenital or acquired immunological disorders, there is persistence of the infection and of the red cell aplasia.

Chapter 15

Haemostasis, Abnormal Bleeding and Anticoagulant Therapy

Learning objectives

- To know the morphology and function of platelets and the relationship between the concentration of platelets in peripheral blood and the extent of abnormal bleeding.
- To know about the diseases associated with (i) a failure of platelet production and (ii) a shortened platelet lifespan, especially autoimmune (idiopathic) thrombocytopenic purpura (ITP).
- To know the main sequence of events in the coagulation pathways.
- To understand normal fibrinolysis and the principles of fibrinolytic therapy.
- To know the principles underlying the prothrombin time (PT), activated partial thromboplastin time (APTT) and thrombin time.
- To know the principles of investigation of a patient suspected of having a haemostatic defect.
- To know the mode of inheritance, clinical presentation, method of diagnosis and principles of treatment of haemophilia, factor IX deficiency and von Willebrand's disease (VWD).
- To know the effects of vitamin K deficiency and liver disease on the clotting mechanisms.
- To know the alterations in the haemostatic and fibrinolytic mechanisms associated with disseminated intravascular coagulation (DIC) and the causes of DIC.
- To understand the principles of anticoagulant therapy with unfractionated and low molecular weight heparin and warfarin and to know about the laboratory control of such therapy.
- To be aware of the natural anticoagulant mechanisms in blood and some of the prethrombotic states (thrombophilia).

Lecture Notes: Haematology, by NC Hughes-Jones, SN Wickramsinghe, CSR Hatton © 2008 Blackwell Publishing, ISBN: 9781405180504

Normal haemostasis

The cessation of bleeding following trauma to blood vessels results from three processes: (i) the contraction of vessel walls; (ii) the formation of a platelet plug at the site of the break in the vessel wall; and (iii) the formation of a fibrin clot. The clot forms within and around the platelet aggregates and results in a firm haemostatic plug. The relative importance of these three processes probably varies according to the size of the vessels involved. Thus, in bleeding from a minor wound, the formation of a haemostatic plug is probably sufficient in itself, whereas, in larger vessels, contraction of the vessel walls also plays a part in haemostasis. The initial plug is formed almost entirely of platelets but this is friable and is subsequently stabilized by fibrin formation.

Classification of haemostatic defects

The action of platelets, the clotting mechanism and the integrity of the vascular wall are all closely related in the prevention of bleeding. However, it is convenient to consider that abnormalities in haemostasis resulting in bleeding arise from defects in one of four processes:

1 A deficiency of platelets (the commonest cause).
2 An abnormality in the clotting mechanism (the second commonest cause).
3 Abnormal platelet function.
4 Vascular abnormalities.

A clinical distinction can frequently be made between bleeding due to clotting defects and

145

bleeding due to a diminished number of platelets. Patients with clotting defects usually present with bleeding into deep tissues, that is muscles or joints. On the other hand, patients with a deficiency of platelets usually present with superficial bleeding, that is, bleeding into the skin and from the epithelial surfaces of the nose, uterus and other organs. Haemorrhages into the skin include petechiae, which are less than 1mm in diameter (Fig. 15.1) and ecchymoses, which are larger than petechiae and vary considerably in size (Fig. 15.2). A further useful clinical distinction is that bleeding usually persists from the time of injury in the case of platelet deficiency, since platelet numbers are inadequate to form a good platelet plug, whereas in clotting defects the initial bleeding may cease in normal time as platelet plugs are readily formed, but as a consequence of the failure to form an adequate clot the platelet plug is not stabilized by fibrin formation and subsequently disintegrates, resulting in a delayed onset of prolonged bleeding. The clinical distinction is by no means complete, as deep-seated haemorrhage is sometimes found in platelet deficiency and, on the other hand, superficial bleeding may occur in clotting defects.

Petechial haemorrhages and ecchymoses and bleeding from other sites may occur when the number of platelets falls below 50×10^9/L. At levels between 20 and 50×10^9/L, petechiae, ecchymoses and nose bleeds are the commonest symptoms, but below 20×10^9/L, gross haemorrhage (melaena, haematemesis, haematuria) becomes increasingly common. However, there is a great deal of variation in the relationship between the platelet count and haemorrhage in individual patients.

Platelets

Morphology and lifespan

Platelets are discoid, non-nucleated, granule-containing cells (2–3μm in diameter) that are formed in the bone marrow by the fragmentation of megakaryocyte cytoplasm. Their concentration in normal blood is 160–450 $\times 10^9$/L.

The plasma membrane of a platelet contains glycoproteins (GPs) that are important in the interaction of platelets with subendothelial connective tissue and other platelets. These include GP Ia, which binds to collagen; GP Ib, which binds to von Willebrand factor (VWF); and GP IIb/IIIa, which binds to fibrinogen. The platelet membrane is extensively invaginated to form a surface-connected canalicular system through which the contents of platelet granules are released. Another intracellular membrane system known as the dense tubular system is rich in calcium, phospholipid-bound arachidonic acid, phospholipase A_2 (which mobilizes arachidonic acid), cyclooxygenase and thromboxane synthase, and is the main site of prostaglandin and thromboxane synthesis. The platelet also contains contractile microfilaments, an equatorial band of microtubules involved in maintaining its normal discoid shape and two main types of ultrastructurally identifiable

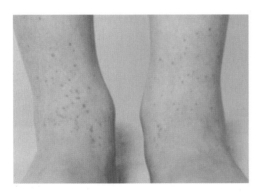

Figure 15.1 Multiple pin-point haemorrhages (petechiae) on the legs of a patient with idiopathic thrombocytopenic purpura (ITP).

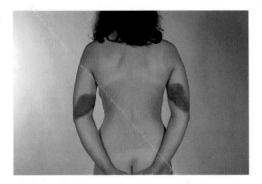

Figure 15.2 Large ecchymoses on both the upper arms of a woman with ITP.

granules. The α-granules, which are the most numerous, contain platelet factor 4 (heparin-neutralizing factor), platelet-derived growth factor (which stimulates mitosis in vascular smooth muscle cells), VWF and fibrinogen. The contents of the dense granules (δ-granules) include adenosine triphosphate (ATP), adenosine disphosphate (ADP), 5-hydroxytryptamine (which causes vasoconstriction) and calcium.

The lifespan of the platelet has been determined by labelling platelets *in vitro* with radioactive chromium (^{51}Cr) and studying their fate after reinjection into the circulation; it is of the order of 10 days.

Physiology

The main function of platelets is the formation of a haemostatic plug at sites of damage to vascular endothelium. First the platelets stick to exposed subendothelial collagen and microfibrils. Adhesion is potentiated by VWF present in plasma. VWF has binding sites for GP Ib on the platelet and for the microfibrils and can thus cross-link platelets to microfibrils. Within 1–2 s of adhesion, platelets change their shape from a disc to a more rounded form with spicules which encourage platelet–platelet interaction (aggregation) and they also release the contents of their granules (platelet release reaction). The most important substance released is ADP. The platelets are also stimulated to produce the prostaglandin, thromboxane A$_2$, from arachidonic acid derived from the cell membrane: thromboxane A$_2$ is an important mediator of the platelet release reaction. The release of ADP and thromboxane A$_2$ causes an interaction of other platelets with the adherent platelets and with each other (secondary platelet aggregation), thus leading to the formation of a platelet plug (primary haemostasis). On the surface of activated platelets, GP IIb/IIIa undergoes a conformational change to provide binding sites for fibrinogen, which plays a role in linking platelets together to form aggregates. Anionic platelet membrane phospholipids are also exteriorized, providing a procoagulant surface on which important reactions of the coagulation

pathway take place. Prostacyclin released by endothelial and vascular smooth muscle cells inhibits platelet aggregation and may thus limit the extent of the platelet plug. Whereas thromboxane A$_2$ is a potent vasoconstrictor, prostacyclin is a powerful vasodilator.

At the site of injury, tissue factor (TF) is expressed and a TF–VIIa complex initiates the formation of a fibrin clot within and around the platelet plug (secondary haemostasis). The anionic phospholipids exposed on the surface of aggregated platelets allow binding of the vitamin K-dependent proteins (factors II, IX and X) and the cofactors V and VIII, thus considerably enhancing the speed of the clotting reaction on and around the platelet surface. Platelets are also responsible for the contraction of the fibrin clot once it has been formed.

Tests of platelet function

Bleeding time

The bleeding time is estimated by making small wounds in the skin of the forearm after applying a blood pressure cuff to the upper arm and inflating it to 40 mmHg; the average time that elapses until bleeding ceases is then measured. The wounds are three punctures made with a lancet in the method of Ivy, or one or two short incisions in the various template methods; the depth of the wound is standardized. The normal range depends on the method and is 2–4 min with the Ivy method. Since the wound only damages small vessels, haemostasis is mainly dependent on the formation of a platelet plug and hence the bleeding time is prolonged either when platelet numbers are reduced or when platelet function is impaired. It is almost always normal in the presence of clotting defects.

When platelet function is normal, there is a good correlation between the platelet count and the bleeding time. Bleeding times are not prolonged until the platelet count has fallen to 100×10^9/L. Below that value, there is a progressive and proportional prolongation in bleeding time, the time lengthening from the normal average of about 3 min to reach about 30 min as the platelet count falls to 10×10^9/L. Below 10×10^9/L, bleeding times may be prolonged to 1 h or more.

On the other hand, when platelet function is impaired, bleeding times are longer than might be expected from platelet numbers (e.g. in uraemia, in von Willebrand's disease (VWD) and after the ingestion of aspirin). The greatest value of the bleeding time is in detecting impaired platelet function in individuals with a normal platelet count. The bleeding time is being replaced by an *in vitro* estimation of primary haemostasis using a machine called PFA 100.

Other tests

A large number of *in vitro* tests of platelet function have been described. The most commonly used tests study the aggregation of platelets following the addition of substances such as ADP, adrenaline, thrombin, collagen or ristocetin to platelet-rich plasma. Aggregation causes a decrease in optical density and the test is performed using special equipment capable of continuously recording optical density.

Thrombocytopenic and non-thrombocytopenic purpura

'Purpura' is the collective term for bleeding into the skin or mucous membranes. Patients with purpura can be separated into those with low platelet counts (thrombocytopenic) and those with normal platelet counts (non-thrombocytopenic). The non-thrombocytopenic group can be subdivided into those patients who have qualitative platelet defects and a larger group who have vascular abnormalities. The latter is a miscellaneous group and contains congenital disorders such as hereditary haemorrhagic telangiectasia (Fig. 15.3) and the Ehlers–Danlos syndrome and acquired diseases such as Henoch–Schönlein purpura (allergic purpura), scurvy, purpura senilis and the purpura of infectious diseases. A type of purpura, purpura simplex ('simple easy bruising'), which may also be due to a vascular abnormality, is a common benign condition causing frequent spontaneous bruising of the legs (and no other bleeding symptoms) that affects otherwise healthy females of

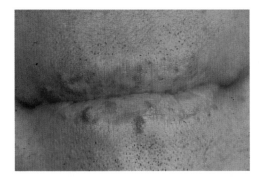

Figure 15.3 Vascular malformations (reddish purple) on the lips of a patient with hereditary haemorrhagic telangiectasia; such lesions are found throughout the body and increase in number with advancing age. This rare condition is inherited as an autosomal dominant characteristic and may lead to recurrent gastrointestinal haemorrhage and chronic iron deficiency anaemia.

child-bearing age. This diagnosis should only be made after excluding other bleeding disorders.

Causes of thrombocytopenia

The mechanisms leading to thrombocytopenia are:

1 A failure of platelet production by the megakaryocytes.
2 A shortened lifespan of the platelets.
3 Increased pooling of platelets in an enlarged spleen.

The distinction between the first two of these possibilities can be made by assessing the number of megakaryocytes in a marrow aspirate or trephine biopsy of the marrow.

The causes of thrombocytopenia are given in Table 15.1.

Failure of platelet production

If megakaryocytes are few or absent, it may be assumed that platelet production is at fault. The bone marrow smears may also reveal other features that indicate the nature of the disease if evidence has not already been obtained from the peripheral blood. Thus, there may be a generalized aplasia of the bone marrow (aplastic anaemia) or a selective decrease in megakaryocytes caused by certain drugs

Table 15.1 Some causes of thrombocytopenia.

Failure of platelet production
Aplastic anaemia (p. 140)
Drugs, alcoholism
Viruses
Myelodysplasia
Paroxysmal nocturnal haemoglobinuria (p. 46)
Bone marrow infiltration (carcinoma, leukaemia,
lymphoma, myeloma, myelofibrosis, storage diseases
including Gaucher's disease, osteopetrosis)
Megaloblastic anaemia due to B$_{12}$ or folate deficiency
Hereditary thrombocytopenia (e.g. thrombocytopenia
with absent radii, grey platelet syndrome, Bernard–
Soulier syndrome, Wiskott–Aldrich syndrome)

Shortened platelet survival
Immune
Autoimmune (idiopathic) thrombocytopenic
purpura
Secondary autoimmune thrombocytopenic purpura
(SLE and other collagen diseases, lymphoma, chronic
lymphocytic leukaemia, HIV infection)
Drugs, alcoholism
Infections (viral, bacterial or parasitic)
Post-transfusion purpura
Neonatal alloimmune thrombocytopenia
Thrombotic thrombocytopenic purpura (most cases)
and haemolytic uraemic syndrome
Non-immune
Disseminated intravascular coagulation (p. 162)
Increased splenic pooling

(e.g. chlorothiazides, tolbutamide), alcoholism and certain viruses (e.g. Epstein–Barr virus, measles, varicella, cytomegalovirus). (Shortened platelet survival mediated through immunological mechanisms is frequently more important than failure of platelet production in the pathogenesis of thrombocytopenia in viral infections.) Another cause of reduced platelet production is marked infiltration of the marrow by malignant cells (e.g. in leukaemia, lymphoma, myeloma and carcinoma) or by fibrous tissue. Reduced platelet production may also occur in patients with normal or increased numbers of megakaryocytes when there is ineffective megakaryocytopoiesis, as in severe vitamin B$_{12}$ or folate deficiency or in myelodysplastic syndromes.

Shortened platelet survival

If the megakaryocytes in the marrow are numerous, then the thrombocytopenia is usually due to an excessive rate of removal of platelets from the peripheral circulation. In most cases the destruction results from autoantibodies attached to the platelet surface and the disease is termed autoimmune (idiopathic) thrombocytopenic purpura (ITP). Occasionally it is due to intravascular platelet consumption due to: (i) DIC; or (ii) interaction with damaged small blood vessels (microangiopathic thrombocytopenia) as in thrombotic thrombocytopenic purpura (TTP) or the haemolytic uraemic syndrome.

Autoimmune (idiopathic) thrombocytopenic purpura (ITP)

ITP is characterized by petechiae (Fig. 15.1), bruising (Fig. 15.2), spontaneous bleeding from mucous membranes and a reduction in the platelet count (without neutropenia or, usually, anaemia). The disease presents in both an acute and chronic form. About 60% of patients with chronic ITP have IgG autoantibodies in their plasma and on their platelets that result in a shortened lifespan due to premature destruction in the spleen. The antibodies are usually directed against the platelet GP IIb/IIIa or Ib. It is thought that acute ITP is caused by immune complexes rather than by platelet autoantibodies. However, there is evidence that autoantibodies against the platelet GP IIb/IIIa and Ib are also present in some patients with this condition. The platelet lifespan is shortened in ITP, often reduced to about 1–2 days or less (e.g. 2 h) compared to the normal lifespan of 10 days. In approximately 30% of patients the destruction takes place only in the spleen, and in the rest it also occurs in the liver.

Clinical features
Acute ITP: This is seen at all ages but is most common before the age of 10 years. Two-thirds of patients give a history of a common childhood viral infection (e.g. upper respiratory tract infection, chicken pox, measles) 2–3 weeks preceding the purpura. Platelet counts are often less than

20×10^9/L. In most patients the disease runs a self-limiting course of 2–4 weeks but in approximately 20% it becomes chronic, that is lasts more than 6 months. The disease is almost always self-limiting when there is a history of preceding infection. The mortality is low, the main danger being intracranial bleeding.

Chronic ITP: This occurs mainly in the age period 15–50 years; it has a higher incidence in women than in men. The chronic form is usually not severe and mortality is low; platelet counts are usually between 20 and 80×10^9/L. Spontaneous cures are rare and the disease is characterized by relapses and remissions. About one-third of the patients with chronic ITP have petechiae and ecchymoses as the only presenting signs. The remainder also have bleeding from the following sites in decreasing order of frequency: nose, gums, vagina (menorrhagia) and gastrointestinal and renal tracts. Cerebral haemorrhage occurrs in about 3%. As a general rule the spleen is not palpable.

Diagnosis

Children with the appropriate clinical features, acute thrombocytopenia and an otherwise normal blood count (i.e. no evidence of acute leukaemia) may be diagnosed as having acute ITP without bone marrow aspiration. The diagnosis of chronic ITP is also based on clinical features and the exclusion of other causes of thrombocytopenia and may not require marrow aspiration. In ITP, bone marrow megakaryocytes are normal or increased in number (up to 4- or 8-fold) and increased in size. An absence or reduction of megakaryocytes rules out the disease. A marrow aspiration also serves to exclude other causes of thrombocytopenia, such as aplastic anaemia, leukaemia or marrow infiltration by carcinoma cells, lymphoma cells or myeloma cells. Thrombocytopenia is sometimes the first sign of systemic lupus erythematosus (SLE). Thrombocytopenia due to drugs must also be excluded.

Treatment

Acute ITP: Over 80% recover without any treatment. Corticosteroids are widely used; they increase the platelet count and so reduce the duration of thrombocytopenia. High doses of intravenous immunoglobulin (Ig) cause a rapid increase in the platelet count and are administered, with or without corticosteroids, to children with severe thrombocytopenia or life-threatening haemorrhage.

Chronic ITP: Treatment is usually not needed in patients with platelet counts above $30–50 \times 10^9$/L who have no significant spontaneous bleeding. High-dose corticosteroid therapy increases the platelet count to more than 50×10^9/L and, usually, more than 100×10^9/L in two-thirds of patients with chronic ITP. Adults are often started on prednisolone 60 mg/day and the dosage reduced gradually after a remission is achieved, or after 4 weeks. However, in only a third of patients who initially have a complete remission, is the remission long lived.

Splenectomy should be considered if the response to corticosteroids is poor, the minimum dose of corticosteroid required to prevent bleeding is unacceptably high or a patient relapses after responding to corticosteroids. About 75% of the patients respond fully to splenectomy, usually within 1 week. However, 10–15% of complete responders will relapse after an interval.

Azathioprine or cyclophosphamide can be used in patients who fail to respond to splenectomy, in an attempt to reduce antibody formation. These drugs have been reported to be effective in some cases.

High doses of intravenous Ig (e.g. 400 mg/kg/ day for 5 days) have also been found to increase the platelet count to greater than 50×10^9/L in 80% of patients with chronic ITP and to normal values in more than 50%. However, the increase is usually transient; the platelet count returns to pretreatment levels in 2–6 weeks. Ig probably acts by interfering with platelet destruction by inhibiting the binding of the Fc portion of the IgG antibodies on the platelet surface to Fc receptors on macrophages.

Other treatments that have been used in refractory patients include danazol, antiD Ig and rituximab.

Secondary autoimmune thrombocytopenic purpura

An autoimmune thrombocytopenia may precede other manifestations of SLE by several years and may complicate the course of SLE, other autoimmune disorders, lymphoma and chronic lymphocytic leukaemia. Patients infected with the human immunodeficiency virus (HIV) may develop either autoimmune thrombocytopenia or immune thrombocytopenia (caused by immune complexes) long before developing other characteristic features.

Drug-induced immune thrombocytopenia

Certain drugs such as heparin, gold salts, quinine, quinidine, sulphonamides or penicillin cause a shortening of platelet lifespan in a small proportion of recipients by an immunological mechanism. The drug (e.g. quinine or quinidine) binds to the platelet membrane, and antibody formed against the drug–platelet complex combines with platelets that have reacted with the drug but not with normal platelets. Heparin causes moderate or severe thrombocytopenia in 1–3% of recipients by a variation of this mechanism: the drug binds to α-granule-derived platelet factor 4 (PF4) on the platelet surface and the heparin–PF4 complexes act as neoantigens. The resulting immune complexes combine with the Fc receptors of platelets causing platelet activation and, in some cases, thrombosis.

Increased splenic pooling

A normal spleen contains within its microcirculation about 30% of all the blood platelets; the platelets in the splenic pool exchange freely with those in the general circulation. The splenic platelet pool increases with increasing splenic size so that in patients with moderate to massive splenomegaly it may account for 50–90% of all blood platelets, thus causing thrombocytopenia. Another factor contributing to the thrombocytopenia in patients with splenomegaly is an increase in plasma volume (p. 48).

Other immune thrombocytopenias

In the rare condition known as *post-transfusion purpura*, severe thrombocytopenia develops 5–8 days after a transfusion, as a result of the destruction of the recipient's platelets. Platelet-specific alloantibodies are present in the serum but the explanation for the destruction of the patient's own platelets is unclear.

Transient but potentially serious *neonatal alloimmune thrombocytopenia* may occur in babies of healthy mothers. The mother forms IgG alloantibodies against a fetal platelet-specific antigen lacking in the mother's platelets and inherited from the father; these antibodies cross the placenta and damage fetal platelets (analogous to haemolytic disease of the newborn, p. 177).

TTP and haemolytic uraemic syndrome

In healthy individuals a VWF-cleaving protease (ADAMTS 13) cleaves the Tyr 842-Met 843 peptide bond in VWF to produce the characteristic multimer profile. In the absence of the protease, ultra-large VWF multimers are released that lead to platelet aggregation and the disease known as 'thrombotic thrombocytopenic purpura' (TTP). Familial relapsing TTP is due to the autosomal recessive inheritance of a deficiency of the protease. Sporadic TTP is due to an IgG antibody against the protease. This is a serious illness characterized by fever and widespread arteriolar platelet thrombi leading to fragmentation of red cells, thrombocytopenia, neurological symptoms and renal impairment. The haemolytic uraemic syndrome is a similar disorder affecting infants, young children and the elderly in which the arteriolar thrombi are predominantly formed in the kidneys; in some patients, the disease follows a bout of diarrhoea caused by verotoxin-producing *Escherichia coli* or shiga toxin-producing *Shigella dysenteriae*. Shiga toxin stimulates the release of ultra-large VWF multimers from endothelial cells and inhibits the cleavage of such multimers by ADAMTS 13 thereby causing multimer-mediated adhesion of platelets to endothelial cells.

Abnormalities of platelet function

These must be suspected in any patient with non-thrombocytopenic purpura. An acquired defect of platelet function is found after aspirin ingestion and after therapy with sulphinpyrazone (a competitive inhibitor of cyclo-oxygenase) or dipyridamole (Persantin). Aspirin has a moderate effect on the bleeding time: 2h after the ingestion of 600mg of aspirin, the bleeding time rises above the normal range in 30% of subjects and may be as long as 20 min. This prolongation is sufficient to provoke abnormal bleeding in certain people and aspirin is contraindicated in those with bleeding disorders. Aspirin acts by irreversibly acetylating cyclo-oxygenase and this inhibits thromboxane A_2 synthesis with a subsequent reduction in platelet aggregation. The effect of a single dose of aspirin can be detected for 1 week (i.e. until most of the platelets present at the time of taking the aspirin have been replaced by newly formed platelets).

Another antiplatelet drug, clopidogrel, acts by irreversibly blocking the ADP receptor (P2Y12) on the platelet cell membrane thereby inhibiting secondary platelet aggregation and the cross-linking of platelets by fibrin.

Various abnormalities of platelet function may also be found after treatment with other drugs such as some non-steroidal anti-inflammatory drugs (e.g. indomethacin or ibuprofen), penicillin, cephalosporins, dextrans, and heparin (high doses) and after the consumption of alcohol.

Other causes of an acquired abnormality of platelet function include chronic myeloproliferative disorders (p. 127), myelodysplastic syndromes, paraproteinaemias (e.g. myeloma or Waldenström's macroglobulinaemia) and uraemia.

Platelet transfusions

It is often possible to raise the platelet count temporarily by platelet transfusions. The main indication for platelet transfusion is severe haemorrhage caused by: (i) thrombocytopenia due to diminished platelet production or DIC; or (ii) abnormal platelet function. Transfusion may also be indicated in a patient with thrombocytopenia or defective platelet function prior to surgery (p. 176). Another indication for platelet transfusion is thrombocytopenia (platelets $<50 \times 10^9$/L) in patients receiving massive blood transfusions (p. 171); blood stored for 48 h has virtually no viable platelets. When thrombocytopenia results from excess destruction caused by platelet antibodies, the response to transfusion is poor. Platelets are transfused as platelet concentrates and should be given within 5 days of withdrawal from the donor (p. 176). In order to prevent *spontaneous* haemorrhage, platelet counts need only be maintained above $10–20 \times 10^9$/L since severe bleeding is rare above this level.

Normal coagulation mechanism

The mechanisms involved in the clotting cascade were elucidated in the period 1950–1970, largely by the work of R.G. MacFarlane and his colleagues. The essential feature of the cascade is the presence of a number of steps activated in sequence. Each step is characterized by the conversion of a proenzyme into an enzyme by the splitting of one or more peptide bonds, which brings about a conformational change in the molecule and reveals the active enzyme site.

The clotting sequence is initiated *in vivo* by tissue factor (TF) exposed on the surface of activated endothelial cells and leucocytes and on most extravascular cells in an area of tissue damage (Fig. 15.4). TF binds to activated factor VII, forming TF–VIIa complexes; the mechanism of activation of factor VII is unclear. The TF–VIIa complexes bind and activate factors IX to IXa and X to Xa. Factor IXa activates factor X. Factor Xa then attaches to the platelet surface and acts on prothrombin (factor II) to generate small amounts of thrombin (factor IIa). This pathway of thrombin generation is rapidly suppressed by tissue factor pathway inhibitor (TFPI). If formed in sufficient quantity, the small amounts of thrombin activate factors VIII,

---

Inherited disorders of platelet function

These are very rare and include:

1 Bernard–Soulier syndrome (autosomal recessive inheritance) in which there is a deficiency of glycoprotein Ib in the platelet membrane and there are giant platelets.
2 Glanzmann's thrombasthenia (autosomal recessive inheritance) in which there is a deficiency of glycoprotein IIb/IIIa in the platelet membrane and platelets are normal in morphology and number.
3 δ-storage pool disease (dense granule deficiency).
4 Grey platelet syndrome (α-granule deficiency).
5 Defects of thromboxane synthesis, including cyclo-oxygenase deficiency and thromboxane synthase deficiency.

Extrinsic pathway:

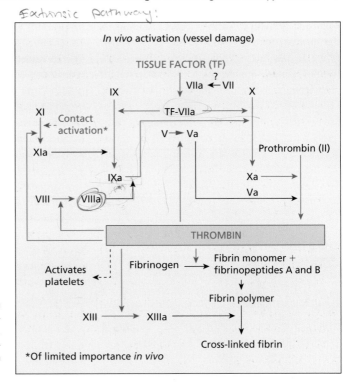

In vivo activation (vessel damage)

TISSUE FACTOR (TF)

Figure 15.4 Pathways involved in fibrin generation after the activation of coagulation *in vivo* by TF. The suffix 'a' denotes the enzymatically active form of each coagulation factor.

V and XI and platelets. Factor XIa converts more factor IX to IXa. Factor VIIIa enhances the activity of factor IXa formed by the action of TF–VIIa complexes and factor XIa on factor IX and markedly amplifies the conversion of factor X to Xa and, consequently, the generation of thrombin from prothrombin which is augmented by factor Va. Thrombin splits two small negatively charged peptide fragments (fibrinopeptides A and B) from fibrinogen (factor I), thus removing repulsive forces from the molecule and allowing the remainder to polymerize and form the fibrin fibre. Finally, factor XIIIa, generated by the activation of factor XIII by thrombin, stabilizes and strengthens the fibrin polymers by forming covalent bonds between the fibrin chains (glutamine–lysine bridges). Calcium is required at several stages in the coagulation sequence. The reactions involving factors IXa, VIIIa and X to form Xa (tenase reaction) take place mainly on the exposed phospholipids on the surface of platelets; the rate of reaction at the surface is considerably higher than that in solution. Hence bleeding in thrombocytopenia results from a

failure of the clotting cascade as well as the lack of a platelet plug.

The extent of thrombin generation is limited by a number of natural anticoagulant mechanisms. Thrombin binds to thrombomodulin on the endothelial cell surface and the resulting complex activates protein C (PC) to activated protein C (APC), which inactivates factors Va and VIIIa in the presence of a cofactor protein S. In addition, free thrombin is directly inactivated by the circulating inhibitor, antithrombin (AT), after the latter binds to heparans on endothelial cells.

Previous *in vitro* studies indicated that there are two pathways or systems present within the coagulation cascade: an intrinsic system, all the components of which are in the plasma, and an extrinsic system consisting of TF, factor VII, factor X (with V as the cofactor), factor II and factor I. The sequence of action of factors in the intrinsic system were considered to be XII, XI, IX (with VIII as the cofactor), X (with V as the cofactor), II and I, as illustrated in Fig. 15.5. The clotting sequence was initiated *in vitro* by activation of factor XII.

Following limited activation, factor XII converts the plasma protein prekallikrein to kallikrein which in turn activates factor XII fully to XIIa. Another plasma protein, high molecular weight kininogen, is a non-enzymatic accelerator of these interactions. Factor XIIa then acts on XI to form the active enzyme XIa. This is not the major pathway of the initiation of coagulation *in vivo* as shown by the absence of a bleeding tendency in people with an inherited deficiency of factor XII. The intrinsic/extrinsic system model remains valuable in understanding laboratory tests for blood coagulation (Fig. 15.5).

Six of the synonyms for the factors are still in general use and should be known. They are: antihaemophilic globulin, VIII; Christmas factor, IX; prothrombin, II; thrombin, IIa; fibrinogen, I; and fibrin, Ia.

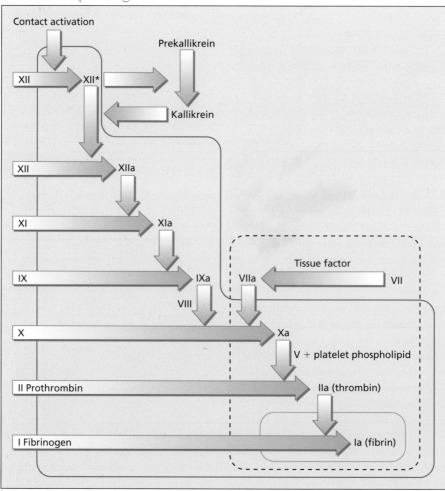

Figure 15.5 The sequence of reactions between the initiation of coagulation *in vitro* by contact activation of factor XII and fibrin formation. The suffix 'a' denotes the enzymatically active form of each coagulation factor. The coagulation factors involved in three basic tests of coagulation are shown within the boxes. Red line — activated partial thromboplastin time; interrupted black line — prothrombin time; blue line — thrombin time.

The fibrinolytic mechanism

The complex mechanism for producing fibrin is counterbalanced by a mechanism for the enzymatic lysis of clots (Fig. 15.6). The dissolution of the fibrin into fibrin-degradation products (FDPs) is carried out by the proteolytic plasma enzyme plasmin. Plasmin is present in the plasma in an inactive form, plasminogen, which is synthesized in the liver; plasminogen binds to fibrin and is converted to plasmin mainly by fibrin-bound tissue plasminogen activator (t-PA) which is synthesized and released by the injured vascular endothelium. Small amounts of plasmin are also generated from plasminogen by urokinase which is produced mainly by renal cells but also other cell types such as endothelial cells. There may also be a limited activation of plasminogen by factors XIa and XIIa and kallikrein. Bradykinin, which is released from high molecular weight kininogen by the action of kallikrein, is a powerful stimulator of t-PA release. The plasma contains two physiological inhibitors of t-PA known as plasminogen activator inhibitor-1 (PAI-1) and PAI-2. Activated protein C (p. 165) inactivates PAI-1 and thereby stimulates fibrinolysis.

Plasmin is not specific for fibrin but can also break down other protein components of plasma, including fibrinogen and the clotting factors Va and VIIIa, and thus the following mechanism is present to confine the activities of plasmin to fibrin. When fibrin is formed, t-PA and plasminogen are specifically adsorbed onto fibrin; the t-PA–fibrin complex has a high affinity for plasminogen and converts it to plasmin, which digests the fibrin to which it is adsorbed. Under normal conditions, any plasmin released from the fibrin into the circulation is immediately inactivated by combining with the liver-derived plasma inhibitors, α_2-antiplasmin and α_2-macroglobulin. In this way, generalized break down of fibrinogen and other proteins does not occur.

Urokinase is the physiological activator of plasminogen present in urine and many secretions; it is produced by epithelial cells of renal tubules and of glandular tissue (e.g. mammary gland ducts). Available thrombolytic drugs include urokinase and recombinant t-PAs as well as non-physiological activators, such as streptokinase, derived from certain streptococci and anisoylated plasminogen–streptokinase activator complex (APSAC). Recombinant t-PAs (alteplase, reteplase and tenecteplase) and streptokinase are the most frequently used drugs and are administered intravenously for the treatment of early acute myocardial infarction. Thrombolytic drugs may also be useful in other types of thrombosis.

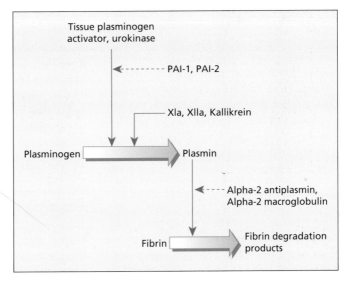

Figure 15.6 The fibrinolytic mechanism. The orange arrows indicate conversion, the continuous red arrows indicate activity, and the broken arrows indicate inhibition. *Note*: PAI-1 — plasminogen activator inhibitor-1.

Tests for clotting defects

There are three basic tests that are widely used:

1 The *activated partial thromboplastin time* (APTT) (e.g. kaolin–cephalin clotting time), which estimates the activity of factors XII, XI, IX, VIII, X, V, II and fibrinogen (the 'intrinsic system') (Fig. 15.5).
2 The *prothrombin time* (PT), which estimates the activity of factors VII, X, V, II and fibrinogen (the 'extrinsic system') (Fig. 15.5).
3 The *thrombin time* (p. 163), which is prolonged when there is an inherited or acquired deficiency of fibrinogen, or an inherited or acquired abnormal fibrinogen molecule (dysfibrinogenaemia) or in the presence of heparin or raised levels of FDPs (Fig. 15.5).

It is evident from Fig. 15.5 that deficiencies of factors X, V, prothrombin (factor II) or fibrinogen will cause prolongations of both the APTT and PT. Patients with liver disease or DIC who have acquired deficiencies of several factors show prolongation of both the APTT and PT. Patients with acquired deficiencies of factors II, VII, IX and X (vitamin K-dependent factors) resulting from treatment with coumarin drugs or from vitamin K deficiency (p. 161) also have a prolonged APTT and PT. The PT is more sensitive than the APTT in detecting these deficiencies because of the short half-life of factor VII. In the small group of patients with congenital defects of one of the clotting factors, 80–90% have haemophilia (factor VIII deficiency), about 10–20% have factor IX deficiency, and only about 1% have deficiencies of one of the other eight factors. Thus, in practice, in almost all the congenital deficiencies the APTT is prolonged and the PT is usually normal. By determining both the APTT and the PT, it is therefore possible to obtain information as to where the defect lies.

Activated partial thromboplastin time

There is a wide range in the time taken for venous blood to clot in a glass tube at 37°C. This wide range in the whole blood clotting time is due to two variables. First, activation of factor XII by the glass surface is variable and depends on such factors as the type of glass. Second, there is a variation in the coagulation-potentiating activities supplied by the platelets, as platelet numbers vary considerably between individuals. The variation due to these two factors can be substantially abolished by the addition of kaolin and a phospholipid (partial thromboplastin). Kaolin provides a maximal stimulus for factor XII activation and the phospholipid acts as a platelet substitute. The test is simple to carry out. Citrated plasma is obtained and to this is added a mixture of kaolin and phospholipid followed by calcium, and the time taken for the mixture to clot is measured. Prolongation of the clotting time is often due to a deficiency of factors VIII and IX (provided that a deficiency of factor X onwards has been excluded by a normal PT) and the test is sufficiently sensitive to detect deficiencies of both these factors when their concentration is reduced to 30% or less of the normal value; that is, it will detect the mild haemophiliacs who only have severe bleeding after minor surgical procedures. A prolonged APTT may also be due to lupus anticoagulant (p. 166) and factor XII deficiency.

If the APTT is prolonged, it is possible to confirm the diagnosis of either factor VIII or IX deficiency if plasma is available from known cases of haemophilia and factor IX deficiency. Thus, if the addition of plasma known to be deficient only in factor VIII does not shorten the clotting time of the sample from the patient under investigation, then the patient must also have a deficiency of factor VIII. Specialized tests are also available for measuring fairly precisely the levels of factor VIII and IX, expressed as a percentage of the normal value; these tests should always be carried out in appropriate cases.

Prothrombin time

The test used to measure the integrity of the extrinsic system is the one-stage PT. This test is carried out by adding tissue thromboplastin derived from brain (TF, factor III) together with calcium to citrated plasma. Reference to Fig. 15.5 shows that TF and factor VII (actually the TF–VIIa complex) initiates coagulation by activating factor X to Xa and hence prolongation of the PT results from deficiencies of I, II, V, VII and X. The PT is thus a misnomer as deficiency of at least five factors affects the test and prothrombin deficiency alone must be gross before the PT is prolonged. The test is chiefly sensitive to deficiencies of factors V, VII and X. A deficiency of platelets does not affect the PT.

When measuring the PT and APTT, it is necessary simultaneously to determine the clotting time using a lyophilized control plasma. This is because there are always small differences in the activities of the reagents that are used.

When the PT is used for the control of oral anticoagulant therapy, the results are expressed as the international normalized ratio (INR). This is derived from the PT ratio (i.e. the patient's PT: mean normal PT) and a factor determined for each thromboplastin reagent by comparing its activity against an international reference preparation. The value of using the INR is that the same therapeutic ranges apply irrespective of the source of thromboplastin.

Congenital coagulation disorders

Blood clotting abnormalities can be conveniently divided into two categories, congenital defects and acquired defects. This section deals with those that are present from birth.

There is a group of patients who complain of excessive bleeding, either spontaneous or following trauma, usually starting early in life, and who frequently have a family history of a similar condition. These patients usually have one of three diseases: haemophilia, factor IX deficiency or VWD.

Haemophilia (factor VIII deficiency, haemophilia A)

The term 'haemophilia,' first used by Schönlein in 1839, was applied to a lifelong tendency to prolonged haemorrhage found in males and dependent on the transmission of a sex-linked abnormal gene. During the decade 1950–1960, it was found that there are in fact two diseases

within the group of patients who, on clinical and genetic grounds, had been diagnosed as having haemophilia: patients with factor VIII deficiency and those with factor IX deficiency. The term haemophilia has been retained for factor VIII deficiency, as this is the more common deficiency; the terms 'factor IX deficiency', 'haemophilia B' or 'Christmas disease' (after the name of the first patient) are used for the other disease.

Genetics, prevalence and biochemistry

Deficiency of factor VIII results from an abnormality in the factor VIII gene, which is very large (186 kilobases, 26 exons) and lies at the tip of the long arm of the X-chromosome. Various abnormalities in the nucleotide sequence of this gene have been identified in about half the cases of haemophilia, ranging from single-point mutations to large deletions. Half of all severe cases are due to an inversion involving intron 22. The disease is almost entirely confined to males (XY) since the normal X-chromosome in heterozygous females is almost always capable of bringing about adequate factor VIII production. The prevalence of this disorder is about one per 10,000 males. Females with haemophilia have been observed extremely rarely and these are either homozygotes for the abnormal gene or are heterozygotes in whom the normal X-chromosome has not produced sufficient quantities of factor VIII due to lyonization. Daughters of males with haemophilia are obligatory carriers of the gene, since they must inherit the abnormal X-chromosome. Sons, on the other hand, are always normal, since they inherit the Y-chromosome. A female with a genetic defect on one X-chromosome will transmit the disease to half her sons, and half her daughters will become carriers. Patients suspected of having haemophilia should be carefully questioned for a history of a bleeding disorder occurring in the relations on the maternal side as opposed to the paternal side. There is a steady spontaneous mutation rate of the gene responsible for factor VIII production, since approximately one-third of all haemophiliacs have no family history of the disease and this has been corroborated from studies on the genomic DNA.

The factor VIII molecule is a protein with a molecular weight of 8×10^4 daltons. In the plasma, factor VIII is only found complexed with VWF, which acts as a carrier and prolongs its plasma half-life. The factor VIII coagulant activity can be measured biologically by its ability to act as a cofactor to factor IXa (see Fig. 15.5); the VWF can be measured by reaction with specific antibodies. Although factor VIII coagulant activity is greatly depressed in haemophilia, the amount of VWF is within normal limits.

Detection of carriers and antenatal diagnosis

Female carriers on average have half the clotting activity per unit of VWF compared to normal. Discrimination, however, is not perfect and in about 10% of carriers the ratio between the clotting activity and VWF content falls within the normal range; thus, those with abnormal ratios can definitely be said to be carriers, but putative carriers with normal ratios cannot be definitely assured that they do not have the abnormal gene. Genetic mutational analysis allows carriers to be identified with better accuracy and is the method of choice today.

Prenatal diagnosis of haemophilia can be made by analysis of fetal DNA or blood. DNA can be obtained either by chorionic villus sampling between 9 and 12 weeks of gestation or by amniocentesis between 13 and 16 weeks. The presence or absence of the abnormal gene can be established either directly using DNA probes for specific defects or indirectly by RFLP (restriction fragment length polymorphism) analysis. Fetal blood sampling is done between 18 and 20 weeks. Factor VIII levels are determined in the fetal plasma either on the basis of immunological reactivity or coagulation activity.

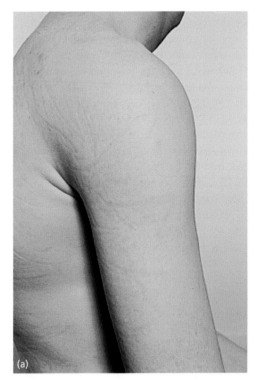
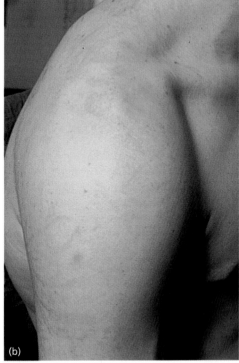

Figure 15.7 Haemarthrosis of the shoulder joint in a patient with haemophilia A.

Table 15.2 The frequency of bleeding sites in 207 haemophiliacs.

Lesion or operation	Percentage
Haemarthroses	79
Muscle haematomas	15
Haematuria	
Epistaxes	
Gastrointestinal bleeding	Each about 1–2
Dental extraction	Total 6
Major surgery	

Source: From Rizza (1977) *Br. Med. Bull. 33*, 225–30.

Clinical features

The characteristic clinical feature of severe haemophilia is the occurrence of spontaneous bleeding into the joints (Fig. 15.7) and less frequently into the muscles; these two sites account for about 95% of all bleeds requiring treatment (Table 15.2). The presenting symptom is pain in the affected area and this can be very severe. Haemophiliacs rapidly become expert at diagnosing the onset of haemorrhage in its earliest stages, allowing treatment to be initiated at a time when it can be most effective. If not properly treated, bleeding into joints results in crippling deformity. The knees, elbows and ankles are most commonly affected. Haematuria, epistaxis and gastrointestinal bleeding are less common. Intracranial bleeding is the most common cause of death from the disease itself (i.e. discounting deaths from HIV infection — see below), accounting for 25–30% of all such deaths; only about one-half of the affected patients have a history of trauma.

The severity of bleeding and mode of presentation is related to the level of plasma factor VIII; this relationship is shown in Table 15.3. The severity of the disease often remains constant throughout a family.

Because of treatment with HIV-contaminated factor VIII concentrates between about 1978 and 1985, over 50% of patients with severe haemophilia in the USA and Europe became HIV-positive; many of these have died of the acquired immune deficiency syndrome (AIDS). In addition, virtually all haemophiliacs have been infected with hepatitis C virus (p. 173) due to treatment with non-virally inactivated factor concentrates.

Table 15.3 The relation between plasma factor VIII levels and severity of bleeding.

Factor VIII level (units/100 mL)	Bleeding symptoms
50	None
25–50	Excessive bleeding after major surgery or serious accident (often not diagnosed until incident occurs)
5–25	Excessive bleeding after minor surgery and injuries
1–5	Severe bleeding after minor surgery (sometimes spontaneous haemorrhage)
0	Spontaneous bleeding into muscles and joints

Source: From Rizza (1977) *Br. Med. Bull. 33*, 225–30.

Diagnosis

The possibility of haemophilia is suggested by the finding of a normal PT and a prolonged APTT. Confirmation can be obtained by showing that the addition of plasma from a known case of factor VIII deficiency to the patient's plasma does not correct the clotting defect whilst the addition of normal plasma does, or confirmation can be obtained by a specific assay of factor VIII coagulant activity. The combination of a normal PT and a prolonged APTT is most often caused by lupus anticoagulant (see p. 166).

Treatment

Treatment should be given at the earliest sign of spontaneous or post-traumatic bleeding. It should also be given prophylactically if any type of operation is contemplated. Treatment consists of intravenous injections of virucidally treated plasma-derived high-purity factor VIII concentrate or recombinant factor VIII preparations to maintain plasma factor VIII coagulant activity to between 5% and 100% of normal, depending on the severity of the injury or extent of the proposed surgical procedure. In general, the more extensive the bleeding or degree of trauma, the larger the dose of factor VIII concentrate that is required. HIV has been virtually eliminated from currently used plasma-derived factor VIII preparations by using donors who do not have HIV antibodies and by employing one or more virucidal methods (e.g. heating the lyophilized product at 80°C, heating in solution at 60°C or adding a solvent detergent mixture during the manufacturing process).

Since the half-life of factor VIII in the plasma is about 12h, this factor has to be injected twice a day. Frequent assays of factor VIII levels in the plasma may be necessary to ensure that the concentration is being maintained at the appropriate level.

Approximately 5–10% of haemophiliac patients who are injected with factor VIII, usually on 9–15 occasions, develop antibodies which inhibit its functional activity. In these patients, the antibody may be swamped with large amounts of human factor VIII or porcine factor VIII concentrates. However, the latter can only be used for a short time, since antibodies to these molecules develop rapidly. Haemorrhage in patients with high-titre inhibitors may require treatment with 'bypassing agents' such as recombinant factor VIIa or FEIBA (factor eight inhibitor bypassing activity – i.e. a plasma-derived activated prothrombin complex concentrate), which activate the coagulation cascade below the level of factor VIII.

The administration of factor VIII may be avoided in mild to moderate haemophilia by using the vasopressin analogue desmopressin (DDAVP), which causes a temporary increase in factor VIII and VWF by provoking the release of these factors from endothelial cells. DDAVP is used intravenously, subcutaneously or intranasally. The antifibrinolytic drug tranexamic acid should be administered with DDAVP as the latter also causes release of t-PA from the endothelium.

Freeze-dried factor VIII concentrates can be stored at 4°C and can be injected in adequate amounts in a small volume. This has made it possible for many patients to be treated at home, sometimes by self-administration, thus allowing factor

VIII to be injected as soon as symptoms appear. Such early therapy results in both rapid cessation of bleeding and rapid recovery. As an extension to this, many severely affected boys receive regular prophylactic treatment with factor VIII.

Factor IX deficiency (haemophilia B, Christmas disease)

The differentiation of factor IX deficiency from haemophilia due to a lack of factor VIII was first made by Biggs and colleagues in 1952. The clinical features and inheritance of factor IX deficiency are identical to those in factor VIII deficiency. Factor IX deficiency affects about one in every 50,000 males (i.e. it is less frequent than factor VIII deficiency). The factor IX gene is located on the long arm of the X-chromosome, is much smaller than the factor VIII gene (containing eight exons) and has been fully sequenced. Mutations in this gene have been found in virtually all cases of factor IX deficiency.

The APTT is prolonged and the PT normal. The diagnosis can be made by assay of the factor IX level. Factor IX concentrate or recombinant factor IX is available and should be administered intravenously as soon as spontaneous or post-traumatic bleeding starts. Factor IX has a longer half-life in the plasma (24h) than factor VIII and hence can be given at less frequent intervals. It has been found that home treatment with factor IX as soon as bleeding starts considerably reduces the need for hospital care.

Von Willebrand's disease

This is the most common inherited bleeding disorder, with a prevalence of 0.8–2%, which is considerably greater than that of factor VIII deficiency. It was described by von Willebrand in 1926 as occurring in several families on islands in the Baltic (Åland Islands). It differs from haemophilia in that the defect is not sex linked but is usually inherited as an autosomal dominant character with varying expression. It is characterized by mild, moderate or severe bleeding. The bleeding results from either a qualitative abnormality or a deficiency of VWF. This factor is a protein with a molecular weight of 2.7×10^5 daltons and exists in the plasma as a variable-sized polymer ranging from a dimer to a molecule containing 50–100 subunits. It has a dual function: first, it is an adhesive molecule which binds platelets to subendothelial tissues; second, it acts as a carrier for factor VIII. The reduction in VWF results in a reduction in factor VIII concentration (usually measured as clotting activity), which may be as low as 5–30% of normal, similar to that found in mild haemophilia. The excessive bleeding in the disease is thus due both to the failure of the platelets to adhere as well as to factor VIII deficiency. An additional finding is that, whereas the antibiotic ristocetin induces platelet aggregation in platelet-rich plasma from normal subjects, it fails to do so in platelet-rich plasma from people with severe VWD. This observation is the basis of a useful laboratory test for the diagnosis of this disease.

The gene for VWF is present on chromosome 12 and analysis of the gene has shown that there is considerable heterogeneity in the genetic defects found in VWD. Some defects result in a reduction in the plasma concentration of structurally normal VWF molecules but others cause different qualitative abnormalities in the VWF molecule. VWD has been divided into three types: in types 1 (most frequent) and 3 there is a partial reduction or nearly complete absence of VWF molecules, respectively, and in type 2 there are qualitative abnormalities.

Most patients are heterozygous for the von Willebrand gene and the extent of bleeding is not great. Spontaneous bleeding is usually confined to mucous membranes and skin and takes the form of epistaxes and ecchymoses, bleeding after dental extraction and menorrhagia. Severe haemorrhage may occur following surgical procedures. Bleeding into joints and muscles is rare except in patients who are homozygous for the defective gene.

The laboratory findings include a prolonged bleeding time, a prolonged APTT, reduced factor VIII clotting activity, reduced levels of VWF and impaired ristocetin-induced platelet aggregation; however, there may be periods when the bleeding time is within normal limits. The prolonged bleeding time distinguishes VWD from haemophilia A and factor IX deficiency.

For mildly or moderately affected patients, desmopressin (DDAVP), which increases plasma levels of both VWF and factor VIII, should be tried before using blood products; it is most effective in type I VWD. In unresponsive patients, intermediate purity factor VIII concentrates that contain VWF and factor VIII are effective in stopping haemorrhage, mainly by correcting the bleeding time but also by increasing factor VIII clotting activity, which continues to increase for many hours after treatment. Alternatively, very high-purity VWF concentrate may be used. High-purity factor VIII concentrates are unsuitable for the treatment of VWD since they contain very little VWF. The antifibrinolytic drug tranexamic acid may be used for treating epistaxis or menorrhagia and in combination with DDAVP- or VWF-containing concentrates to manage dental extractions.

Deficiency of other clotting factors

Single deficiencies of factors other than VIII and IX are very rare, but all possible deficiencies have been found and all except factor XII deficiency give rise to bleeding disorders of varying degrees of severity. The explanation for the absence of excessive haemorrhage in factor XII deficiency is that the activation of the intrinsic pathway can be initiated in the absence of factor XII by the activation of factor IX by factor VIIa of the extrinsic system and the activation of factor XI by thrombin (see Fig. 15.4).

Acquired coagulation disorders

The hepatocytes are the major cell type involved in the synthesis of all the coagulation factors. Hence, severe liver disease may result in bleeding due both to a deficiency of several coagulation factors and to an abnormality in the structure and function of fibrinogen. In addition, liver disease may result in impaired clearance of activated clotting factors or t-PA leading to disseminated intravascular coagulation (DIC) or increased fibrinolysis, respectively.

The final stages in the synthesis of factors II, VII, IX and X (collectively known as the pro-thrombin group or complex) involves a vitamin K-dependent carboxylase, which adds carboxyl (–COOH) groups to the proteins; these groups are necessary for the efficient functioning of the molecules.

The coumarin drugs are vitamin K antagonists and their administration results in only partial carboxylation of the prothrombin group of coagulation factors, which are consequently considerably less active than normal in the clotting cascade. Similar abnormalities are seen in vitamin K deficiency, which may be found in the newborn (haemorrhagic disease of the newborn), in patients with intestinal malabsorption and, since bile salts are required for vitamin K absorption, also in patients with biliary obstruction or biliary fistulae. Examination of Fig. 15.5 shows that except for factor IX, the clotting factors involved in these acquired deficiencies are detected by the PT and that apart from factor VII they are also detected by the APTT. However, as mentioned earlier, the PT is the more sensitive test due to the short half-life of factor VII and, consequently, it is the test employed for monitoring oral anticoagulant therapy and detecting the abnormalities in vitamin K deficiency.

Disseminated intravascular coagulation

DIC describes a process in which there is a generalized activation of the clotting system followed by marked activation of the fibrinolytic system. Acute DIC may be associated with premature separation of the placenta (abruptio placentae), amniotic fluid embolism or shock and may also be seen in certain bacterial infections such as meningococcal septicaemia, where the endotoxin causes damage to monocytes and vascular endothelium. It is a common complication following intravascular haemolysis of red cells after a mismatched transfusion. The syndrome also occurs occasionally after extensive accidental or surgical trauma, particularly following thoracic operations. Chronic DIC is seen when there is retention of a dead fetus as well as in patients with disseminated carcinoma, lymphoma

and leukaemia (especially acute promyelocytic leukaemia). Other clinical associations of DIC include purpura fulminans (following scarlet fever, chicken pox or rubella), brain injuries, extensive burns, liver disease and snake bites.

In those diseases that are associated with DIC, the clotting cascade may be activated in various ways, namely, by the release of TF from damaged tissues, monocytes or red cells; by damage to endothelial cells; and by abnormal activators of coagulation. Activation of the cascade leads to the generation and dissemination of large amounts of thrombin in the circulation, activation of platelets and the formation of intravascular microthrombi. If this is sufficiently extensive, there is a reduction of the concentration of fibrinogen and other clotting factors in the plasma, which impairs haemostatic activity. As a consequence of the fibrin formation, the fibrinolytic mechanism is activated (p. 154) resulting in high concentrations of FDPs and D-dimers. This leads to further haemostatic impairment, since FDPs inhibit fibrin clot formation by interfering with the polymerization of the fibrin monomer. FDPs also interfere with the aggregation of platelets. With continued intravascular coagulation, there is increased expression of thrombomodulin on endothelial cells and the thrombin–thrombomodulin complexes activate protein C; APC inactivates factors Va and VIIIa, further aggravating the haemostatic defect and also inhibits PAI-1, which stimulates fibrinolysis. The end result is generalized haemorrhage due to failure of haemostasis.

The haemorrhagic manifestations may be so severe in acute DIC as to lead to death. They include petechiae, ecchymoses and bleeding from the nose, mouth, urinary and gastrointestinal tracts and vagina. Haemorrhage may also occur into the pituitary gland, liver, adrenals and brain. Although the usual clinical manifestation of acute DIC is haemorrhage, occasionally, the clinical picture is dominated by signs and symptoms of widespread thrombosis and infarction; thrombi are most frequently found in the microvasculature. There may be digital gangrene, adult respiratory distress syndrome, neurological signs and renal failure. Mild hypotension is commonly present in acute DIC and may progress to become more severe and irreversible if not treated in time.

In chronic DIC, the haemorrhagic tendency may be mild or moderate. However, some patients with chronic DIC are asymptomatic because the activation of the clotting and fibrinolytic systems is finely balanced and the production of clotting factors and platelets is sufficiently increased to compensate for their increased consumption.

Diagnosis

This is partly dependent on being aware of the conditions with which DIC is associated. The investigations of value in the diagnosis of acute or chronic DIC are as follows:

1 *The platelet count*: Platelets become enmeshed in the fibrin clots on the vascular endothelium and thrombocytopenia is an early and common sign.
2 *The APTT and the PT*: These are significantly prolonged, due to the depletion of clotting factors, especially in acute DIC.
3 *The fibrinogen concentration*: This is reduced. The best method for the estimation of fibrinogen is based on the time taken for a diluted sample of plasma to clot in the presence of high concentrations of thrombin (the Clauss method).
4 *The thrombin time*: This may be prolonged. When the fibrinogen concentration is normal, estimation of the thrombin time is a useful indication of the presence of excessive amounts of FDPs. The thrombin time is determined by adding low concentrations of thrombin to citrated plasma and measuring the time for the appearance of a clot. In the presence of FDPs, the thrombin time is prolonged due to inhibition of fibrin polymerization.
5 *Estimation of FDPs and the D-dimer assay*: FDPs and D-dimer levels are increased. The presence of FDPs can be detected by rapid immunological tests in which latex particles coated with polyclonal antibody directed against fibrinogen are agglutinated by FDPs present in serum. However, the FDPs assayed may be derived from the degradation both of fibrinogen and intravascular fibrin. This lack of specificity has been overcome by new assays using monoclonal antibodies to the D-dimer fragment generated by plasmin-mediated digestion of the cross-linked fibrin in thrombi.

Treatment

Since the activation of the clotting system is the primary initiating stimulus and fibrinolysis is mainly a secondary phenomenon, treatment is aimed at preventing further coagulation by removal of the initiating cause (e.g. when it occurs in obstetric practice, rapid and non-traumatic vaginal delivery stops the clotting process). Whilst the initiating cause is being dealt with, patients with acute DIC should be supported with transfusions of blood, fresh-frozen plasma and platelet concentrates in order to restore blood volume and to replace clotting factors and platelets.

Anticoagulant drugs

The two most frequently used anticoagulant drugs are heparin and warfarin. Parenteral heparin is used in patients with deep vein thrombosis (DVT) or pulmonary embolism (PE) and is followed by warfarin therapy to reduce the risk of recurrence. The same combination is used in acute anterior transmural myocardial infarction to decrease the possibility of systemic embolism. Subcutaneous heparin is used to reduce the risk of DVT and PE in patients undergoing surgery (especially hip surgery) and in patients with acute myocardial infarction. Heparin does not cross the placenta and is therefore the preferred drug when anticoagulation is required during pregnancy. The oral anticoagulant warfarin is administered usually for 3–6 months, to patients with DVT or PE and after the insertion of xenograft mitral heart valves. Lifelong warfarin therapy is indicated in patients with recurrent venous thrombosis, with rheumatic mitral valve disease complicated by embolism or atrial fibrillation, and with prosthetic heart valves.

Heparin

Standard unfractionated heparin is an acidic mucopolysaccharide (average molecular weight

1.5×10^4 daltons) that has to be administered intravenously or subcutaneously. When administered intravenously, its biological half-life is 1 h. Heparin potentiates the action of AT, a molecule that inactivates the activated serine protease coagulation factors, thrombin (IIa), IXa, Xa and XIa; the greatest effect is on IIa. Low molecular weight heparin (average molecular weight $4–5 \times 10^3$ daltons) is used subcutaneously; it inactivates Xa to a greater extent than IIa and has a longer biological half-life. Two examples of low molecular weight heparins currently in use are dalteparin (Fragmin) and enoxaparin (Clexane).

For the treatment of thrombosis or embolism, standard heparin may be administered as a bolus of 5000 units (70 units/kg) intravenously, followed by a continuous intravenous infusion of 15–25 units/kg/h. Treatment is monitored by performing the APTT, the heparin dosage being altered so as to maintain the APTT at 1.5–2.5 times the normal value although these figures may vary with different APTT reagents. However, the treatment of choice is now low molecular weight heparin given subcutaneously once a day with no monitoring (because of the high predictability of effect when given accordingly to body weight). When a patient on heparin is started on warfarin, there should be a minimum overlap period of 3 days and the heparin should be stopped only when a full warfarin effect is achieved.

Either standard or low molecular weight heparin is administered subcutaneously to prevent venous thrombosis in patients subjected to surgery or in patients with myocardial infarction or when long-term heparin therapy is required. The dosage of standard heparin for prevention of postoperative thrombosis is 5000 units subcutaneously preoperatively followed by 5000 units subcutaneously 12 hourly for 7 days or until the patient is fully mobile. Low molecular weight heparin is administered once daily.

Haemorrhage due to overdosage is managed by stopping the heparin and, if necessary, by giving protamine sulphate intravenously. Side effects include impaired platelet function, heparin-induced thrombocytopenia (HIT) via an antibody-based mechanism (see p. 151), osteoporosis (following long-term use), alopecia and hypersensitivity reactions.

Warfarin sodium

This is a coumarin derivative that is administered orally once a day. As has already been mentioned, it is a vitamin K antagonist and interferes with the carboxylation and hence with the functional activity of factors II, VII, IX and X, protein C and protein S. After the first dose, clotting factor activity is reduced in the order VII, IX, X and II (i.e. the factor with the shortest half-life is reduced fastest and the longest half-life most slowly).

It is customary to prescribe 10 mg warfarin on the first day and to determine the prothrombin ratio (the ratio of the patient's PT to the mean normal PT) and INR (i.e. the prothrombin ratio standardized by correcting for the sensitivity of the thromboplastin used) 16 h later. Subsequent doses are based on the INR. The therapeutic ranges of INR commonly recommended are 2–3 for a first DVT or PE, transient ischaemic attacks, arterial disease, arterial grafts and to prevent systemic embolism in patients with atrial fibrillation, mitral valve disease, myocardial infarction or tissue heart valves. A higher range of 3–4 is used for recurrent DVT or PE, recurrent systemic embolism and for patients with prosthetic heart valves.

There are many possible causes for loss of control of warfarin therapy. These include the simultaneous use of drugs that decrease absorption of vitamin K (e.g. antibiotics or laxatives), reduce binding of warfarin to albumin (e.g. phenylbutazone) or inhibit hepatic microsomal degradation (e.g. cimetidene). Bleeding is controlled by stopping the warfarin and, if serious, also by infusing fresh-frozen plasma and by administering vitamin K (2–5 mg i.v.). In life-threatening haemorrhage, prothrombin complex concentrates can be given to correct the defect rapidly and completely. High-dose vitamin K therapy is followed by a period of resistance to warfarin.

Warfarin crosses the placenta and may cause developmental abnormalities such as chondrodysplasia, microcephaly and blindness. It is therefore contraindicated in the first trimester of pregnancy. It should also not be administered during the last few weeks of pregnancy because of its anticoagulant effect on the fetus and the consequent risk of fetal or placental haemorrhage.

Investigation of a patient with abnormal bleeding

A most important step in the diagnostic process is the taking of a good history from the patient. The physician should ask, amongst others, the following questions: Has the patient ever bled excessively in the past and have any relatives bled excessively? More specifically, has the patient had tonsillectomy, major abdominal or orthopaedic surgery or dental extractions in the past, and if so was there any abnormal bleeding? The relationship between the type of bleeding and the nature of the haemostatic defect has been discussed earlier (p. 145).

The screening tests that are useful in investigating a patient who gives a history of excessive bleeding are the following:

1 A blood count, including a platelet count.
2 Examination of a blood film.
3 The bleeding time.
4 The prothrombin time.
5 The activated partial thromboplastin time.
6 The thrombin time.
7 Fibrinogen assay.

If any of these tests is found to be abnormal, further specialized tests may be necessary. The screening tests do not reliably exclude VWD and, if suspected, specific tests should be done.

Natural anticoagulant mechanisms and the prethrombotic state (thrombophilia)

There are natural anticoagulant mechanisms in the plasma that prevent localized fibrin formation from becoming widespread. The most important molecules involved in these mechanisms are AT, protein C and protein S, all of which are produced in the liver. Inherited or acquired abnormalities of these inhibitors of coagulation may

lead to a prethrombotic state (thrombophilia). This section summarizes the essential information relating to: (i) the congenital deficiency of these factors; (ii) prethrombotic states due to the presence of a specific mutation in factor V (factor V Leiden) or prothrombin (G20210A mutation); and (iii) one acquired prethrombotic state known as the antiphospholipid syndrome.

Antithrombin

This is mainly an inhibitor of thrombin and factor Xa, but it also inhibits factors IXa and XIa and the TF–VIIa complex; its action is markedly potentiated by heparin. Normally some AT becomes activated by binding to endothelial cell-associated heparin sulphate and thus prevents thrombus formation on the endothelium. Congenital AT deficiency is inherited as an autosomal dominant character; its prevalence is about 1 in 1500. There are a number of molecular variants of AT, with different degrees of risk of thrombosis. Heterozygotes (whose AT concentrations are 40–50% of normal) may suffer from recurrent DVT, mesenteric vein thrombosis and PE; the first thrombotic event usually occurs between the ages of 15 and 50 years. Homozygotes are rarely seen, presumably due to fetal wastage.

Protein C and protein S

Two other inhibitors of coagulation are the vitamin K-dependent substances, protein C and protein S. Protein C becomes activated when it reacts with thrombin bound to thrombomodulin, a protein of the endothelial cell membrane. Activated protein C (APC) is a serine protease and degrades factors Va and VIIIa; it also promotes fibrinolysis by inactivating PAI-1 (p. 154). Protein S potentiates the effects of APC.

Some individuals have a hereditary deficiency of protein C, with about 50% of normal levels; these are heterozygotes for a mutation affecting the protein C gene and in one study were found with a prevalence of about 1 per 250. A proportion of such heterozygotes displays the clinical picture seen in inherited AT deficiency but in addition are particularly prone to develop superficial thrombophlebitis, cerebral vein thrombosis and coumarin-induced skin necrosis. Homozygotes for the mutant gene are rare, and those who have virtually no protein C present with purpura fulminans or extensive thrombosis of visceral veins in the neonatal period.

Some heterozygotes for protein S deficiency suffer from recurrent venous thromboembolism. Homozygotes are severely affected and suffer from purpura fulminans in the neonatal period.

The incidence of protein C deficiency in children and adults below the age of 45 years with recurrent venous thrombosis is about 5% and the incidence of protein S deficiency in this group is similar.

Factor V Leiden and APC resistance

An abnormality inherited as an autosomal dominant character confers resistance to the anticoagulant effects of APC and is associated with a familial tendency to DVT. In over 90% of cases, this abnormality results from a mutation in factor V (Arg^{506} → Gln); the mutant factor is poorly degraded by APC. In white Caucasian populations, about 5% are heterozygous for the mutation. Factor V Leiden is found in about 20% of cases of venous thrombosis (first episode). Heterozygotes have a 7-fold increase in the risk of thrombosis and homozygotes a 50-fold increase. Some homozygotes for the factor V Leiden mutation suffer from myocardial infarction at an early age.

Prothrombin allele G20210A

One to two per cent of the population have a G20210A mutation in the 3′ untranslated region of the prothrombin gene that increases prothrombin

levels. This increases the risk for venous thrombosis 4-fold.

The antiphospholipid syndrome

The antiphospholipid antibody syndrome is defined by the presence of antiphospholipid antibodies (either anticardiolipin antibodies or lupus anticoagulant) associated with certain clinical features. Lupus anticoagulant prolongs the results of coagulation tests that depend on phospholipid (e.g. the APTT). Although these antibodies have an anticoagulant effect *in vitro*, they are associated with thromboses *in vivo*. Features of the antiphospholipid syndrome may include recurrent venous thromboses (most commonly DVT of the lower limbs), recurrent arterial thrombosis (most commonly stroke but also myocardial infarction), and recurrent abortions (due to placental thrombosis and infarction). Thrombocytopenia is common. Antiphospholipid antibodies are found in some patients with SLE or other autoimmune disorders as well as in individuals with no other evidence of an immunological abnormality. Recent work on the mechanisms underlying the thrombotic tendency suggests that the relevant antibodies are directed not against phospholipid but against plasma proteins that bind to phospholipid, most commonly β2 glycoprotein I and prothrombin, and phospholipid–protein complexes on endothelial cell surfaces. Some antibodies appear to be directed against APC, protein S, HMWK, factor XII, factor Xa and t-PA. The end result is an imbalance between the procoagulant and anticoagulant systems leading to thromboses. Patients who have suffered a thrombotic event are treated long term with antiplatelet drugs and/or anticoagulants.

Chapter 16

Blood Transfusion and Haemolytic Disease of the Newborn

Learning objectives

- To know about the inheritance of the ABO system, and the type and distribution of associated antibodies.
- To know the distribution and mode of inheritance of the D antigen of the Rh system.
- To know the principles involved in the selection of donor blood of suitable ABO and Rh groups for a recipient, and the principles of the cross-match, including the antiglobulin test.
- To know the hazards of blood transfusion (incompatible blood, pyrogenic and allergic reactions, bacterial infection, citrate toxicity and transmission of disease) and of massive blood transfusion.
- To know how to investigate a patient suspected of receiving an incompatible transfusion.
- To know the basis of blood fractionation and the rationale for the use of specific blood products, including red cells, platelet concentrates, fresh-frozen plasma (FFP) and various factor concentrates.
- To understand the principles of requesting blood for routine surgical procedures.
- To know the pathogenesis, clinical features and the principles underlying the treatment and prevention of haemolytic disease of the newborn (HDN) due to anti-D.
- To know the principles of antenatal care concerned with predicting both the presence and severity of HDN due to anti-D.
- To know the differences between HDN due to anti-D and that due to anti-A and anti-B.

Lecture Notes: Haematology, by NC Hughes-Jones, SN Wickramsinghe, CSR Hatton © 2008 Blackwell Publishing, ISBN: 9781405180504

Blood transfusion

One of the main problems in the transfusion of blood is the avoidance of immunological reactions resulting from the differences in the chemical constituents of the red cells between donor and recipient. Blood groups have arisen because mutations have occurred in the genes controlling the surface constituents of the red cells. These alterations in the surface structures have not usually affected the function of the red cell, but when the red cells of a donor are transfused into a recipient who lacks these surface structures, the recipient treats them as foreign substances and produces antibodies against them. There are 29 major sites on the chromosomes where there are genes responsible for red cell surface constituents and there are over 270 well-recognized phenotypes; each of these sites is responsible for a different blood group system. Although all the systems have given rise to transfusion difficulties (and in fact this is how they have been recognized), only two, the ABO and Rh systems, are of major importance.

ABO system

The ABO system has three allelic genes, *A*, *B* and *O*. The first two genes are responsible for converting a basic substance, H, present in every red cell, into A or B substances, thus converting the cells into groups A or B. The *O* gene has no known effect on the H substance, so that group O red cells simply contain H substance. H substance is a carbohydrate chain combined to lipid or protein in the red cell membrane. A terminal sugar molecule is attached to this chain that determines the antigenic specificity, N-acetylgalactosamine in the case of A antigen and galactose in the case of B antigen. The *A* and *B* genes each code for the two different enzymes (glycosyltransferases) which attach these terminal groups. The *O* gene has no recognized product. The three allelomorphic genes combine in pairs to give six possible genotypes, *AA, AO, BB, BO, AB* and *OO.*

In determining the blood group of a person, it is necessary to distinguish between genotype and phenotype. Genotype refers to the specific genes that the person carries, whereas the phenotype refers to the observed characteristics, that is, the agglutination reactions brought about by the appropriate antibodies. Determination of the ABO blood group of a person is carried out using only two antibodies, anti-A and anti-B, through agglutination reactions. Genotypes can only be determined by family studies (e.g. the genotype *AO* and *AA* cannot be distinguished by agglutinating antibodies and both of these genotypes will be classified as the phenotype A). Thus, only four phenotypes are distinguished, namely A, B, AB and O. As the phenotype A includes the genotypes *AA* and *AO*, it follows that a mating between two people of phenotype A can produce a child of group O, if both parents are genotypically *AO.* The same principle holds for the phenotype B.

The frequency of the ABO groups differs in different populations; in the UK it is approximately: group O, 46%; A, 42%; B, 9%; and AB, 3%.

Substances with antigenic properties closely similar to those of A and B are widely distributed in nature and are found in many animals and bacteria. Absorption of these substances from the gut is presumed to give rise to the production of anti-A and anti-B in the plasma of those who do not possess the substances on their red cells. Because of the presence of these antibodies it is necessary to transfuse blood with the same ABO group as that of the recipient. People of group O were at one time known as 'universal donors.' However, this is a dangerous concept, because group O people have anti-A and anti-B in their plasma, and in a small number of people these antibodies may be very potent so that a unit of group O blood may contain sufficient anti-A or anti-B to react with the recipient's cells and bring about their destruction.

Rh system

The Rh system derives its name from the findings of K. Landsteiner and A.S. Wiener in 1940 that the antibody produced in rabbits by the injection of red cells from the Rhesus monkey would agglutinate the red cells of about 85% of humans (Rh-positive) but not of the remaining 15% (Rh-negative). It was quickly discovered that a similar antibody could also be found in the plasma of humans after blood transfusion and in the plasma of mothers who had given birth to a child with hemolytic disease of the newborn (HDN). Several other antibodies were found in humans that were clearly recognizing antigens within the Rh system and, in 1943, R.A. Fisher put forward the theory that there are three allelomorphic pairs of genes within the Rh system, *C* and *c*, *D* and *d*, *E* and *e*. It was postulated that each gene was responsible for producing a different protein molecule on the surface of the red cell, termed C, c, D, d, E and e. Recent genetic analysis, however, has shown that the genetic structure is more complex in that there are only two genes, *RHD* and *RHCE*. The *RHD* gene is responsible for the production of the D protein, a polypeptide of 417 amino acids lying within the lipid membrane and spanning it 12 times; there is no *d* gene and Rh-negative people are those in whom the *D* gene is absent. The other gene, *RHCE* is responsible for the C, c, E and e antigens similar in structure to the D protein and only differing from it by 35 amino acids. There are four common alleles of this gene, namely *CE, Ce, cE* and *ce* coding for four polypeptides; each protein has two antigen sites, namely, either C and E, or C and e, or c and E, or c and e (both antigenic sites are on the same molecule). Thus, individuals carrying the *CE* and *ce* genes (one on each chromosome) will have C, E, c and e antigenic sites on the surface of their red cells.

People who were labelled as Rh-positive on the old nomenclature have the D antigen on their red cells. Thus, people who are either homozygous *DD*, or heterozygous *Dd*, are Rh-positive. Despite the non-existence of *d*, it is convenient to retain the symbol *d* and the genotype *dd* for Rh-negative people to indicate the absence of *D*. The two genes *RHD* and *RHCE* are on chromosome 1 and lie very close together since no crossing-over has ever been found. Thus they are always inherited as a specific combination, the three most common being *DCe*, *dce* and *DcE*. As one of the chromosomes in each chromosome pair is derived from the father and one from the mother, the final genotype might be *DCe/dce*, which is the commonest combination. Rh-negative blood transfusion donors are always *dce/dce*.

Differentiation of people into the Rh-positive and Rh-negative groups is carried out only with anti-D antibody. Use of an antibody of only one specificity means that homozygous *DD* people cannot be differentiated from heterozygous *Dd* people. However, since all the genes of the Rh system are inherited in specific combinations, determination of the presence or absence of the other antigens (C, c, E and e), especially when combined with family studies, can almost always differentiate *DD* from *Dd*. This assessment is sometimes required to determine whether an Rh-negative mother who has anti-D in her plasma can conceive an Rh-negative child by an Rh-positive father; this can only happen if the father is *Dd*.

Clinically, only the D antigen and anti-D are important. The reason for this is that the D antigen is a much more potent antigen than C, c, E or e. Thus, an Rh-negative person (i.e. *dce/dce*) has over 50% chance of developing anti-D after the transfusion of one unit of Rh-positive blood, whereas the 'c' antigen will only provoke anti-c production in 2% of people lacking this antigen. It is thus important that Rh-negative people receive Rh-negative blood. On the other hand, the risk of immunization after giving Rh-negative blood (*dce/dce*) to an Rh-positive person who lacks the 'c' antigen (for instance whose genotype is *DCe/DCe*) is very small.

Other blood group systems

Other blood group antibodies, which are sometimes a problem during blood transfusion, include the following: anti-K (Kell system), anti-Fy^a (Duffy system), anti-Jk^a (Kidd system) and anti-S (part of the MNSs blood group system). Unless an antibody against one of the antigens in these systems is present in the recipient, there is no need to take these groups into account in selecting donor blood. The chief reason for this is that these antigens are also 'poor' antigens. Thus, compared to the D antigen, their relative potency in stimulating antibody production is 10–1000 times less.

Compatibility

The purpose of cross-matching blood before transfusion is to ensure that there is no antibody present in the recipient's plasma that will react with any antigen on the donor's cells. The basic technique for detecting the antibody (i.e. agglutination of the red cells by antibody) has remained unchanged for over 100 years. Agglutination was first observed in 1869 by A. Creite, a medical student in Göttingen, when he found that the serum of one animal would agglutinate red cells of another species; the fact that the agglutinating agents were antibodies was not discovered until 1890.

Unfortunately, many red cell antibodies are unable to bring about agglutination without additional help, such as proteolytic treatment of the red cells or the use of an antiglobulin reagent (see below). The ability of antibodies to agglutinate untreated red cells depends partly on the molecular structure of the antibody. IgM antibodies (molecular weight 9×10^5 daltons) are large and readily span between adjacent red cells and thus can bring about agglutination. By contrast, the smaller IgG antibodies (1.6×10^5 daltons), which are far more common than IgM, do not usually agglutinate, the main exception being IgG anti-A and anti-B.

Antiglobulin test

The antiglobulin test was first discovered by C. Moreschi in 1908, but was forgotten as it had no practical significance at that time, and was rediscovered by R.R.A. Coombs, A.E. Mourant and R.R. Race in 1945. The basic constituent of an antiglobulin serum is antihuman IgG and is obtained by injecting human IgG into animals. Being bivalent, anti-IgG is able to bring about agglutination of IgG-coated red cells by linking IgG molecules on one red cell with those on an adjacent red cell and thus holding the cells together as agglutinates.

The antiglobulin test can be used in two ways. Firstly, it can be used to detect antibody already on the patient's cells *in vivo*. Red cells are washed to remove the free IgG in the plasma, which would otherwise react with and neutralize the antiglobulin. After washing, antiglobulin serum is added and agglutination takes place (the direct antiglobulin test). Secondly, the test can be used to detect the presence of antibody in serum, as in the cross-matching of blood for transfusion. In this case, serum from the patient requiring transfusion is incubated with red cells from the donor blood. Any antibody present in the recipient's serum that has specificity for antigens on the donor's cells will combine with the latter and, after washing, addition of antiglobulin serum will bring about agglutination (the indirect antiglobulin test).

Procedure for obtaining compatible blood

The ABO and Rh group of the recipient must first be determined by the addition of agglutinating anti-A and anti-B to the red cells and the grouping is checked by determining whether anti-A or anti-B is present in the recipient's serum by adding known group A and B cells. Group A blood always contains anti-B in the plasma, group B blood has anti-A and group O has anti-A and anti-B. The Rh group is determined using an agglutinating IgM anti-D or by using IgG anti-D combined with the antiglobulin test.

Donor blood of the appropriate ABO and Rh group is then selected but before this can be transfused, cross-matching must be carried out, partly to ensure that there have been no errors in the determination of the ABO group of the donor and recipient, and partly to ensure that no other antibodies are present in the recipient that react with the donor's red cells. A search is made for both agglutinating and non-agglutinating antibodies, the latter with the antiglobulin test.

In most transfusion laboratories it is now usual for the sera of all recipients to be screened for the presence of antibodies such as anti-K (Kell), anti-Fy^a (Duffy) and anti-Jk^a (Kidd), using a panel of red cells of known phenotype, whenever time permits. If screening is not carried out, these antibodies will be discovered in the final stages of a cross-matching procedure, using the antiglobulin test.

Blood grouping, antibody screening and cross-matching were initially performed in microtitre plates but many laboratories now use automated machines. A computer system maintains data and checks compatibility and excludes units that may react with clinically significant antibody present in the recipient's serum. The advantage of this system is that it allows rapid availability of blood and reduced manpower.

Rh-negative donor blood is not always available for Rh-negative recipients and the question arises whether it is safe to give Rh-positive blood. Rh-negative males, especially elderly males, may receive Rh-positive blood provided care is taken to search for anti-D if subsequent transfusions of Rh-positive blood are given. In women past the menopause the procedure is less safe because there is always the possibility, admittedly small, that they may have received a primary stimulus with D antigen from an Rh-positive fetus and the anti-D in the plasma may be below a detectable level. Transfusion of Rh-positive blood would then provoke a secondary response of anti-D production leading to a delayed transfusion reaction after a few days. Rh-positive blood must never be given to Rh-negative girls or Rh-negative women of child-bearing age for fear of stimulating anti-D production and thus of producing HDN in a subsequent pregnancy.

Donor blood

Donor blood (approximately 450 mL) is mixed with citrate–phosphate–dextrose-containing adenine (CPD-adenine), a solution found empirically

Table 16.1 Total issues of blood components from the transfusion services of the UK in 2004–2005.

Red cells	2,428,934
Platelets	258,528
Fresh-frozen plasma	313,019
Cryoprecipitate	102,719
Total	3,103,200

Note: One unit = component derived from one blood donation.

to give good preservation of the blood. If the blood is stored at 4°C, 80% of the cells are still viable after 28 days, the remaining 20% being removed from the circulation by the reticuloendothelial system within a few hours of transfusion. After 35 days of storage, the percentage of viable cells falls off fairly rapidly, so that the blood is not used after this period of time. Stored blood has reduced levels of red cell 2,3-DPG (p. 2), but levels return to at least 50% of normal within 24 h of transfusion. When plasma is removed from CPD-adenine blood to prepare FFP (fresh frozen plasma) or plasma products, or platelet and granulocyte concentrates, the red cells may be transfused after storage for up to 35 days either in CPD-adenine or, if all the plasma is removed, in a solution containing saline, adenine, glucose and mannitol (SAG-M). Data on the usage of blood components in the UK are given in Table 16.1.

Transfusion in acute haemorrhage and chronic anaemias

Patients with acute haemorrhage (i.e. loss of red cells and plasma) should be transfused with whole blood or with red cells suspended in SAG-M. If more than 10 units of stored blood have to be transfused within 24 h (massive transfusion), patients may need platelet transfusions and FFP. Plasma-reduced blood with a packed cell volume (PCV) of about 65% or concentrated red cells in SAG-M should be used when patients with a severe chronic anaemia have to be transfused, as such patients have an increased plasma volume and are prone to develop circulatory overload (p. 175). Leucocyte-poor blood, usually prepared

by filtering plasma-reduced blood, is used in patients on a long-term blood transfusion programme or in those who have repeated febrile transfusion reactions due to white cell antibodies. Some countries require all blood products to be leuco-depleted. In the UK concerns that variant Creutzfeldt–Jacob disease (v-CJD) is harboured in white cells has led to this requirement.

Hazards of blood transfusion

Since the appearance of acquired immune deficiency syndrome (AIDS), the attitude of the general public to blood transfusion has completely changed and there is now a demand for transfusion without risks, although this can never be achieved. The hazards of transfusion have to be evaluated in terms of risk analysis and the concept of 'risk tolerance' is the most important aspect. The term 'risk tolerance' was first introduced in a report in relation to nuclear power in the UK but is equally applicable to transfusion. To quote this report 'Tolerability does not mean acceptability. It refers to the willingness to live with risks to secure benefits and in the confidence that it is being properly controlled. To tolerate a risk means that we do not regard it as negligible or something that we might ignore, but rather as something we need to keep under review and to reduce still further if and as we can' (Layfield (1987) *Sizewell B Public Enquiry*, HMSO, London).

The unfavourable reactions to transfusion are either immediate or delayed. Immediate reactions are usually due to pyrogens, allergens, bacteria, circulatory overloading or incompatible blood; delayed reactions are due to the transmission of disease, usually of viral origin.

Serious Hazards of Transfusion Committee

Blood transfusion is generally safe, nevertheless there are serious hazards associated with the administration of blood products. In the UK, all adverse incidents following blood transfusion are reported to the Serious Hazards of Transfusion (SHOT) Committee. The nature of the incidents

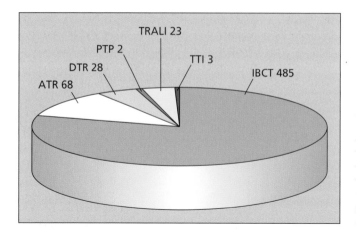

Figure 16.1 Pie chart showing hazards of transfusion in the UK in 2005 ($n = 609$) as reported to the SHOT Committee. *Notes:* TRALI — transfusion-associated acute lung injury; TTI — transfusion-transmitted infection; ATR — acute transfusion reaction; DTR — delayed transfusion reaction; PTP — post-transfusion purpura; IBCT — incorrect blood component transfused.

and the relative frequency reported during 2005 are given in Fig. 16.1.

The commonest error reported to the SHOT Committee is the transfusion of a blood component intended for another patient ($n = 485$) and there were 10 ABO-incompatible transfusions. The main reasons for this are errors in the labelling of blood sample taken for cross-matching and the failure to match the name on the blood pack with that of the recipient.

Whilst labelling errors are common, mistakes happen all the way through the process of ordering, cross-matching and the giving of blood. Most hospitals now have a transfusion committee to implement safety procedures in an attempt to reduce error. Electronic tagging and identification may also help to reduce error.

Haemolytic reactions due to incompatible red cells

The symptoms that are found after a transfusion of incompatible blood depend on whether the transfused cells undergo intravascular lysis or whether they are phagocytosed by the reticuloendothelial system and subjected to extravascular lysis. Intravascular lysis leads to haemoglobinaemia and haemoglobinuria and is almost always due to the action of anti-A or anti-B, which brings about lysis in conjunction with the complement system. Symptoms may appear from a few minutes to several hours after beginning to transfuse

ABO-incompatible blood and may include restlessness, anxiety, fever, chills, flushing of the face, pain in the lumbar region and chest, vomiting and diarrhoea. If the reaction is severe, there is circulatory collapse. These effects result from the release into the plasma of the complement fragments C3a, C4a and C5a, which cause contraction of smooth muscle and degranulation of mast cells. Sometimes, extensive haemorrhage may occur due to disseminated intravascular coagulation (DIC; p. 162), as a consequence of the release of tissue thromboplastin from lysed red cells and hypoxic tissue. There is also about a 10% chance of developing oliguria or anuria; this is probably a consequence of hypotension and DIC.

The immediate treatment of a mismatched transfusion is to promote diuresis with frusemide (furosemide). When deaths do occur, they are usually the result either of severe DIC or of renal failure. The overall mortality following ABO incompatibility is probably of the order of 10%.

When blood transfusion is followed by extravascular destruction of red cells, there are usually only chills and fever occurring one or more hours after the start of the transfusion. The most common antibody causing extravascular destruction is anti-D. This type of incompatibility is almost never followed by renal failure.

Another type of incompatibility is the delayed haemolytic transfusion reaction (DTR). This occurs when a recipient has been previously immunized by transfusion or pregnancy but in whom the antibody in the plasma has become too weak to be identified. Following the transfusion, a secondary immunological response takes place and the antibody titre rapidly rises, bringing about haemolysis, usually about 7 days later. Typically, the patient develops anaemia, fever, jaundice and sometimes haemoglobinuria.

Transfusion-transmitted infections

The risk of transfusion-transmitted infections (TTIs) has declined over the last decade due to the adoption of a number of safety strategies. TTIs accounted for 2% of SHOT between 1997 and 1998 and for only 0.5% in 2005. The majority of TTIs are due to bacterial contamination (p. 175). Other TTIs include hepatitis B (HBV), human T-cell leukaemia virus (HTLV) and human immunodeficiency virus (HIV) infection and hepatitis C (HCV). These infections are not detected in donated blood usually as a result of collecting donations early in the course of an infection before antibody to the virus can be detected. The risk of receiving a unit of infectious blood is less than 1:500,000 for HIV, 1:100,000 for HCV and 1:70,000 for HBV.

Various tiers of safety procedures have been put in place. 'Self-exclusion' is a very important contributor to blood safety. Those donors who are in 'high-risk' categories are asked not to donate, for example recent travel to a tropical country (risk of malarial transmission), a history of intravenous drug abuse, etc. Testing for evidence of HIV, HTLV, HBV and HCV infection in donated blood is a very important aspect of blood product safety. Another important aspect is the use of *pathogen inactivation technology* to inactivate viruses, bacteria, fungi and protozoa. The addition of solvent/detergent will inactivate the lipid envelope of viruses such as HBV, HCV, HIV and HTLV, and others such as Epstein–Barr virus (EBV) and cytomegalovirus (CMV). This process is only suitable for non-cellular components such as factor VIII and intravenous immune globulin. Other methods for inactivation of pathogens include the use of photochemical systems such as psoralen-S59 compounds where, after the addition of the psoralen, the blood product is exposed to high-intensity ultraviolet A light. The latter system may be suitable for platelet concentrates and other cellular products; however, this technology is still largely at the research stage.

HIV and HTLV

HIV-1 is the principal cause of AIDS. The virus is a retrovirus and has the capability of converting its RNA genome into a DNA provirus, which is integrated into the genome of the infected host. The principal route of transmission is by sexual contact; by intravenous drug abuse; by exposure to infected blood products; or from an infected mother to her child during pregnancy, childbirth or breast feeding. Human T-cell leukaemia/lymphoma virus is endemic in certain parts of the world including Japan and Afro-Caribbean countries. Like HIV, HTLV is a retrovirus although it only causes disease in a small proportion of infected patients. Two disorders are recognized in patients carrying this virus, T-cell lymphoma/leukaemia and tropical spastic paraparesis. The virus appears to be transmitted in the same way as HIV. Many countries have compulsory screening programmes for both viruses.

Hepatitis B

HBV is a DNA virus that produces surface protein, hepatitis B surface antigen (HBsAg), which appears in the plasma and can be used for its detection. Transmission causes either acute infection, with subsequent clearance and the development of immunity, or chronic infection with continuing viral replication. Complications include cirrhosis, liver failure and hepatocellular carcinomas. If the screening HbsAg test is positive, confirmatory tests are used to determine the stage of infection (e.g. anti HBc (antibody to hepatitis B core antigen) and anti-HBe (antibody to hepatitis B e-antigen)).

Hepatitis C

HCV is an enveloped RNA virus. Infection causes either acute infection with resolution or chronic persistent infection. The antibody response to

HCV is relatively weak. There are many types of HCV and only a limited number of HCV-specific antigens can be used in screening tests. Donations collected during the 'window period' (i.e. a time during which HCV RNA is present before an immune response) can transmit infections. Therefore, HCV RNA screening of pooled donor samples further increases the safety of blood for transfusion.

Variant Creutzfeldt–Jakob disease

CJD is one of a group of transmissible spongiform encephalopathy disorders. There is a long incubation period and so far no treatment for the progressive, severe damage done to the central nervous system. Rapidly progressive dementia is followed by early death. There have been four likely cases of v-CJD transmission by blood transfusion and concern exists of iatrogenic transmission through blood products. As a precaution, UK blood services exclude anyone with a potential risk of developing v-CJD (i.e. received blood products from or gave blood to individuals who subsequently developed v-CJD) and anyone who has received a blood transfusion since 1980 from donating blood. In addition, all units of blood are leuco-depleted to reduce potentially infected white cells from donors transmitting the disease. There is currently no screening test for v-CJD.

Cytomegalovirus

CMV is a DNA herpes virus present in white cells. The virus is transmitted via respiratory secretions, sexually and during childbirth. The incidence of CMV antibodies varies in different parts of the world from 30% to 80% or more. As with most herpes viruses, the virus persists latently after infection. However, only a small proportion of antibody-positive blood is infective; it is thought that between 1% and 20% of all units of blood have the potential to transmit the virus.

In normal immunocompetent people, the disease varies from a subclinical infection to the appearance of lymphadenopathy and a mild hepatitis. The main danger of CMV infection is in infants and immunocompromised patients and thus prevention of CMV infection is targeted to defined patient groups. Premature neonates of low birth weight born to mothers without anti-CMV antibody are especially at risk. It has been found that 25–30% of such infants developed the infection following transfusion and about 25% of those infected died. Patients receiving bone marrow and solid organ transplants are also at risk (see Chapter 13). Many transfusion centres have established panels of anti-CMV-negative donors specifically for use in these recipients.

Other diseases

Other diseases known to be transmitted by transfusion include syphilis and malaria. The prevention of transmission of syphilis is by serological testing of donors, although this will not demonstrate all those infected since it is possible to have syphilis with negative serological tests. Another factor of importance is the storage of blood at 4°C since spirochaetes do not survive for more than a few days under these conditions. Individuals who have returned from an area where malaria is endemic are not accepted as donors for 1 year, and those who have lived in such an area for a continuous period of 6 or more months are now not accepted in the UK. Brucellosis, babesiosis, Chagas' disease (caused by *Trypanosoma cruzi*), West Nile virus (prevalent in the USA and Canada) and parvovirus B19, which is not inactivated by detergent methods, have also been transmitted by transfusion.

As new diseases emerge from time to time the risk of TTI always remains. It is therefore important that transfusion is only given when essential for survival or quality of life so that benefits clearly outweigh the uncertain risks of TTI.

Transfusion-associated graft versus host disease

Transfusion of viable white cells in blood products can in very rare circumstances lead to transfusion-associated graft versus host disease (GVHD). This invariably fatal disorder can be eliminated by irradiating the blood products (red cells, platelet or plasma) before administration. Most cases have been reported when large volumes of blood have been given to a patient who by chance shares a proportion of histocompatibility antigens with the donor. The donor white cells are not eliminated by immune mechanisms in the normal way; they engraft leading to a rash and bone marrow failure. Patients who have received T-cell cytotoxic chemotherapy such as *fludarabine* must receive *irradiated blood products* as they are at special risk of developing this complication.

Pyrexia due to pyrogens and leucocyte antibodies

Febrile reactions occur during 0.5–1% of transfusions. Reactions due to the presence of pyrogens (soluble bacterial polysaccharides) in the anticoagulant are now extremely uncommon. Most febrile reactions are caused by the presence in the recipient of anti-HLA antibodies or granulocyte-specific antibodies, resulting from immunization during pregnancy or previous transfusions. They usually consist of chills and fever starting 30–60 min after the onset of the transfusion. Such reactions can often be prevented by the administration of an antipyretic or by using leucocyte-poor red cells (p. 171). Since reactions due to pyrogens are now rare, febrile reactions should always suggest the possibility that incompatible red cells or leucocytes have been transfused.

Immediate-type hypersensitivity

Hypersensitivity reactions may occur soon after the transfusion of blood or plasma. The antibodies involved are often unknown but some severe reactions are caused by antibodies against IgA present in recipients who lack IgA and who have previously become sensitized to this immunoglobulin. In mild cases, the only manifestation may be urticarial wheals, erythema, maculopapular rash or periorbital oedema. In the more severe reactions, hypotension may occur; bronchial spasm and laryngeal oedema are rare. Mild reactions probably occur in about 1–3% of transfusions and can be treated with antihistamines.

Severe reactions are very infrequent (1:20,000) and these require the administration of hydrocortisone and adrenaline.

Bacterial contamination

Transfusion of infected blood is rare, but when it does occur it is frequently lethal. Bacterial contamination can occur at several points (contaminated blood bags, donor venepuncture or at the time of transfusion). Bacteria that have been implicated are usually normal skin flora or other ubiquitous organisms. Skin contaminants entering donor blood are usually staphylococci but these are killed off during storage and are only rarely found after 3 weeks. Occasionally, however, gram-negative bacteria enter donor blood and these will grow slowly at 4°C (doubling time about 8 h). In 2–3 weeks at 4°C, growth can be sufficient to cause a lethal reaction. The growth rate of these bacteria is considerably speeded up if the blood is kept at room temperature and the risks of transfusing infected blood can thus be minimized by keeping blood at 4°C until the moment of transfusion. The chief signs of transfusion of infected blood are the rapid onset of pyrexia and circulatory collapse. Haemorrhage due to DIC may occur.

Circulatory overload

Circulatory overload with consequent cardiac failure can easily be brought about by the too rapid transfusion of blood, especially in the elderly and in those who have been severely anaemic for some time. The first signs are dyspnoea, a dry cough, crepitations at the lung bases and a rise in jugular venous pressure. The transfusion must be stopped and venesection may be necessary. The risk of overload can be minimized in patients with severe anaemia by administering frusemide (furosemide), giving concentrated red cells (p. 171) and restricting the rate of transfusion to 1 mL/kg body weight per hour. If the patient is only mildly anaemic and has normal cardiac function, 1 L can be safely transfused over a 5-h period. This is about one drop per second with the standard giving sets.

Citrate toxicity

Citrate toxicity may develop and can cause death if large volumes of stored blood have to be given very rapidly. It is due to the reduction in ionized calcium in the patient's plasma. The signs are gross skeletal muscle tremors and prolongation of the QT interval in the electrocardiogram. If more than 2 L are given every 20 min then each litre should be accompanied by 1 g of calcium gluconate.

Other hazards

Stored blood is deficient in platelets and labile coagulation factors, V and VIII (e.g. blood stored for 5 days contains no platelets and only 30% of the normal factor VIII concentration). Therefore, massive blood transfusions lead to moderate thrombocytopenia and abnormalities in the prothrombin time and activated partial thromboplastin time. When massive blood transfusions are complicated by a haemorrhagic state, bleeding may be controlled by the administration of platelet concentrates and, if the prothrombin time is prolonged by 5 s or more, by fresh-frozen plasma (FFP).

As each unit of blood contains about 250 mg of iron, the administration of frequent transfusions over several years results in a marked accumulation of iron in the body (iron overload) and progressive widespread tissue damage. The iron overloading can be prevented or limited by treatment with desferrioxamine subcutaneously via a pump.

Procedure in the case of transfusion reactions

It is not always easy to diagnose the type of transfusion reaction by the symptoms. Allergic reactions are obvious and, if mild, only require antihistamines. Symptoms occurring within 20 min of starting a transfusion are often due to red cell incompatibility or infected blood and clearly the transfusion must be stopped. It is the occurrence of rigors and fever after 30–60 min that causes difficulty in the diagnosis, since some of these reactions are due to bacterial pyrogens and some are due to leucocyte or red cell incompatibility. In these patients with delayed symptoms, the transfusion should be temporarily stopped, the blood being replaced with saline, and the patient warmed. If symptoms do not rapidly disappear, the transfusion should be abandoned and the reaction investigated further. Fortunately, reactions of this type, due to incompatibility, are only rarely fatal.

Investigation of a transfusion reaction due to incompatibility

There are two questions to answer after a suspected transfusion of incompatible blood: first, has destruction of red cells in fact taken place and, second, which antigen–antibody system was involved. Immediately after the transfusion has been stopped, a blood sample is obtained from the recipient and the plasma is examined for the presence of free Hb and the bilirubin concentration is estimated. A urine sample is also examined for the presence of Hb. If incompatible cells are still present in the recipient's circulation, their presence can often be detected by serological methods. Thus, the presence of group A cells in a group O patient can be detected by the addition of anti-A, which will agglutinate only A cells in the sample.

The ABO and Rh groups of both the recipient and donor are checked and a cross-match repeated using the serum obtained from the recipient prior to transfusion. These tests will reveal whether the incompatibility is within the ABO system or whether it involves the D antigen of the Rh system. If the ABO and Rh(D) groups are compatible, but the cross-match shows the presence of an antibody, the specificity of the antibody can be identified by further testing against a panel of red cells of known blood group specificity. The remains of the donor blood in the pack after every transfusion should be kept at 4°C for 48 h so that any adverse reaction can be adequately investigated.

Platelet and granulocyte concentrates

Platelet concentrates are prepared either from freshly donated units of blood or by using intermittent-flow or continuous-flow cell separators that separate platelets from blood and return the rest of the blood to the donor. They may be stored at 22°C for about 5 days. Platelet concentrates are indicated when there is clinically significant bleeding due to thrombocytopenia or a qualitative platelet defect. They should also be given prophylactically in patients with transient severe thrombocytopenia due to chemotherapy. Prior to surgery, platelet concentrates are used to obtain a platelet count between 50 and 100 $\times 10^9$/L, depending on the nature and severity of the proposed surgical procedure.

Granulocyte concentrates are prepared using cell separators or by pooling buffy coats from donated blood and may be beneficial in patients with intractable bacterial infections associated with severe neutropenia who do not respond to antibiotics.

Haemolytic disease of the newborn

HDN is a consequence of the passage of fetal red cells across the placenta resulting in the immunization of the mother to blood group antigens that she does not possess. The antibodies produced are subsequently transferred back across the placenta (only those of the IgG class are transferred) and react with the fetal red cells causing their destruction. Transplacental haemorrhage most commonly occurs at the time of labour and thus it is usually only in subsequent pregnancies that babies are affected. Before the advent of prophylactic therapy, almost all the cases (93%) were due to the anti-D of the Rh system, 6% were due to other antibodies within the Rh system and only about 1% due to antibodies in other blood group systems. Without treatment, the mortality rate of affected infants is about 20%, but the antenatal prediction of the disease, together with the introduction of treatment by exchange transfusion has considerably reduced this value. Approximately 60% of affected infants require an exchange transfusion, and, in the best hands, efficient treatment results in the survival of about 95% of all those who are born alive. During the decade 1958–1968, the disease resulted in about 300–400 neonatal deaths each year in the UK and an approximately equal number were stillborn. The introduction during 1968 of prophylactic injections of anti-D into the mother immediately after labour to prevent active immunization greatly reduced the incidence, and, by the turn of the century, only about 10–20 deaths occurred each year in the UK due to anti-D; 3–4 deaths resulted from the presence of other antibodies.

Haemolytic disease due to anti-D

The aetiology of HDN was first elucidated by Levine and colleagues in 1941. A mother who had given birth to an affected infant was transfused with her husband's blood and this was followed by a transfusion reaction. It was correctly surmised that the mother had been immunized by a fetal antigen that had been derived from the father. The Rh blood group system was also discovered during this period and it was soon ascertained that the maternal antibody in this mother was anti-Rh, now known as anti-D.

Small numbers of fetal cells can occasionally be found in the maternal circulation throughout pregnancy, especially during the third trimester, but the main transplacental passage occurs at the time of labour; the volume of the haemorrhage is usually less than 5 mL but occasionally may exceed 50 mL. There is evidence that the greater the number of fetal cells in the circulation, the greater the chance of developing antibodies. The relationship between the total amount of fetal red cells in the maternal circulation immediately after labour and the incidence of immunization of mothers 6 months later is shown in Table 16.2.

In the UK population, about 17% of the women are D-negative but, before the advent of preventive therapy, only about 6% of all D-negative women became immunized to the D antigen. The reason for this is 3-fold: firstly, only 83% of fathers carry the D antigen and a substantial number of these are heterozygous, hence having only a 50% chance of transmitting the *D* gene; secondly, the amount of fetal red cells crossing the placenta is often insufficient to initiate immunization; and thirdly, only about 60–70% of Rh-negative mothers

Table 16.2 The relationship between the number of fetal red cells in the maternal circulation after labour and the subsequent immunization of the mother.

Estimated number of fetal red cells (mL)	Incidence of immunization (%)
0	3.7
0.02	4.5
0.04	10.3
0.06–0.08	14.6
0.1–0.2	18.7
0.22–0.78	21.1
>0.8	23.5

Source: From Clarke (1968) *Lancet* **ii**, 1–7.

are able to respond to the D-antigen by producing significant amounts of anti-D.

It is very unusual for the first-born child to be affected with HDN, the incidence being slightly less than 1% of all Rh-negative mothers who have no history of transfusion or abortion. The reason for this is that it is only occasionally that significant numbers of fetal red cells cross the placenta sufficiently early in pregnancy to stimulate anti-D production before the child is born.

If the fetal red cells in the mother after labour bring about a primary immunization, antibody may be found within the following 6 months. In about half the cases, however, antibody concentrations do not rise sufficiently high for anti-D to be detected at this time. During a subsequent pregnancy with an Rh-positive fetus, it only requires a few fetal red cells crossing the placenta early in pregnancy in order to provide a secondary stimulus to anti-D production, which can usually be detected by the 28th week but sometimes may not appear until the last few weeks of pregnancy.

Clinical features

There is a very great variation in the severity of the disease in a child. At one end of the scale there are infants who are not anaemic at birth and who never become jaundiced. However, the Hb concentration of these infants may fall abnormally rapidly after birth and values as low as 6 g/dL may be found up to 30 days later. All neonates with antibodies on their red cells (positive direct

antiglobulin test) should therefore be followed up for a month after birth.

Moderately severely affected babies may or may not be anaemic at birth, but the rate of red cell destruction is such that jaundice develops within a few hours. Jaundice is not seen at the time of birth since prior to this the bilirubin is excreted by placental transfer. Within 48–72 h of birth, the plasma bilirubin may rise to 350–700 μmol/L. The rate of rise of plasma bilirubin is governed partly by the rate of red cell destruction and partly by the degree of maturity of the bilirubin excretory mechanism, that is, on the state of development of glucuronyl transferase. As a result of the poor development of the excretory mechanism for bilirubin in many infants, it is quite common for a child with a cord Hb within the normal range (lower limit 13.5 g/dL) to become severely jaundiced. The danger associated with a high bilirubin level is kernicterus resulting from damage to the basal ganglia of the brain, with a clinical picture characterized by spasticity, arched back and death from respiratory failure. Those that survive usually have a subnormal intelligence.

Severely affected babies become so anaemic that they develop cardiac failure and are either stillborn or die shortly after birth, although those with mild cardiac failure can be resuscitated by exchange transfusion. Apart from anaemia, the characteristic feature of these children is oedema. The stillbirth rate is approximately 15% of all fetuses with haemolytic disease and death may occur from the 20th week onwards.

The presentation of HDN due to anti-D has changed enormously after prophylactic anti-D therapy was introduced.

Management of mother and child

The ABO and Rh blood groups of all pregnant mothers are determined early in pregnancy, and all those who are Rh-negative are examined for the presence of anti-D at 12 weeks and again at 28 weeks. This latter time is chosen because if anti-D is present, this is also the optimum time for carrying out amniocentesis for the antenatal determination of the severity of the disease.

A method of predicting the severity of the disease with certainty would be very valuable since a considerable proportion of affected infants are stillborn and about half of these deaths occur after the 36th week of pregnancy, but unfortunately assessment is still unreliable. Attempts at prediction take into account the amount of anti-D in the mother's plasma (high concentrations are associated with increased severity), the previous history of affected infants (severity runs in families) and examination of the bilirubin concentration in the amniotic fluid, which gives an indication of the extent of haemolysis. None of these is a reliable guide when taken singly, but prediction is improved when all three are considered together. Ultrasound examination is useful to detect fetal hydrops and Doppler ultrasound of the middle cerebral artery is now the screening test to detect fetal anaemia. If anaemia is confirmed by ultrasound guided fetal blood sampling, intrauterine transfusion (usually i.v.) is commenced at about 18 weeks. Since about half the total numbers of stillbirths occur after the 36th week of pregnancy, induction at 36 weeks reduces the incidence of stillbirth and if complications are detected earlier, the baby may have to be delivered even at 32 weeks.

When anti-D is present in the mother's plasma, cord blood is obtained at delivery and the presence of antibody on the red cells confirmed by the antiglobulin test (the strength of the reaction is no guide to severity). If the cord Hb concentration is below the normal lower limit of 13.5 g/dL, an exchange transfusion with Rh-negative blood is required. If the Hb concentration is within the normal range, the decision to give an immediate exchange transfusion rests on the cord bilirubin concentration. Some paediatricians perform an exchange transfusion if this is above 70 μmol/L but others have different criteria. Even if the cord Hb concentration is normal, death can still occur from kernicterus if the ability to excrete bilirubin is poorly developed. About half the patients with Hb concentrations within the normal range require an exchange transfusion because of a rising bilirubin concentration despite optimal phototherapy.

Prevention of Rh immunization

It is possible to bring about a very considerable reduction in the incidence of Rh immunization by giving injections of anti-D intramuscularly to an Rh-negative mother within 72 h of giving birth to an Rh-positive child. In May 2002 the National Institute for Clinical Excellence (NICE) recommended that all non-sensitized RhD-negative women should also be given anti-D prophylaxis at 28 and 34 weeks of pregnancy. Those RhD-negative mothers that carry RhD-negative babies who, of course, are not at risk of RhD haemolytic disease and would therefore not require prophylactic anti-D may now be detected by determining the Rh status of the baby using the tiny amounts of fetal DNA in maternal plasma employing molecular techniques; however, this is usually not done. The injected anti-D combines with the fetal red cells in the mother's circulation and brings about their destruction in the spleen. The precise mechanism by which the suppression of immunization is brought about is not known, but it is assumed that splenic destruction of fetal red cells must divert D antigen on the surface of the cells away from those sites in the immunological system where antibody production is initiated.

Anti-D should be given to all Rh-negative women having an abortion, amniocentesis or external version or who have suffered abdominal trauma in order to prevent primary immunization against the D antigen. It is also possible to use anti-D to prevent primary immunization when a large amount of Rh-positive blood has been inadvertently transfused.

Haemolytic disease due to anti-A and anti-B

Haemolytic disease due to anti-A or anti-B is almost entirely confined to group A and B infants born to group O mothers, since it is mainly group O mothers who have anti-A and anti-B of the IgG class. ABO HDN (of all grades of severity) affects about one per 150 of all births. With the successful prophylaxis of HDN due to anti-D through the use of anti-D injections, clinically significant disease is now more frequently due to anti-A or anti-B or to antibodies other than anti-D within the Rh system, or rarely, to involvement of other blood group systems. Unlike HDN due to anti-D, ABO HDN may be seen in the first pregnancy. ABO HDN is usually very mild; stillbirths do not occur, severe anaemia is uncommon and the child rarely requires treatment by exchange transfusion. Phototherapy is usually sufficient to reduce bilirubin levels. A consistent finding is the presence of spherocytes in cord blood. In certain parts of the world, ABO HDN is even more common than in the UK. This may in part result from the high concentrations of IgG anti-A and anti-B in such populations.

Chapter 17

Basic Haematological Techniques and Reference Ranges

This chapter deals with the principles underlying the measurement of the most commonly determined haematological values. The significance of a measurement made on a patient is judged by comparison with a reference range determined from a population of reference subjects. Such reference subjects must be carefully defined with respect to relevant variables such as state of health, age, sex and race.

Haemoglobin concentration and the blood count

Until about three decades ago, the haemoglobin concentration per decilitre of blood (Hb), packed cell volume (PCV), white cell count (WBC), red cell count (RBC) and platelet count were all determined by manual methods. Today, in all diagnostic laboratories of the developed world, basic haematological parameters are measured not by manual methods but by semiautomated or fully automated electronic blood counting machines. Current fully automated machines provide at least the following data on every sample analysed: WBC, Hb, RBC, PCV, mean cell volume (MCV),

mean cell haemoglobin (MCH), mean cell haemoglobin concentration (MCHC) and platelet count. However, two of the manual methods, namely, the cyanmethaemoglobin method for haemoglobin estimation and the Wintrobe haematocrit method (with a correction for trapped plasma), continue to be the reference methods.

Haemoglobin concentration

Manual method

The estimation of Hb is dependent on its property of absorbing light in the yellow–green region of the visible spectrum. The blood is diluted with a solution containing potassium cyanide and potassium ferricyanide that converts all types of haemoglobin (oxyhaemoglobin, reduced haemoglobin, methaemoglobin and carboxyhaemoglobin) into the stable cyanmethaemoglobin compound. The optical density of the solution is then measured using a photoelectric colourimeter or spectrophotometer; the instrument is calibrated using a cyanmethaemoglobin standard. Hb is expressed as grams of haemoglobin per decilitre of whole blood.

The accuracy of any particular estimate, as carried out in a routine laboratory, is probably of the order of ±5%. The chief sources of error are failure to mix the blood adequately before sampling

Lecture Notes: Haematology, by NC Hughes-Jones, SN Wickramsinghe, CSR Hatton © 2008 Blackwell Publishing, ISBN: 9781405180504

and inaccurate dilution. The reference ranges for the Hb at different ages are given on p. 16.

Automated method

In most fully automated blood-cell counters, the haemoglobin level is estimated by an adaptation of the cyanmethaemoglobin method.

Estimation of PCV

Glass tubes with an internal diameter of about 3 mm (Wintrobe haematocrit tubes) or much smaller (microhaematocrit tubes) are filled with anticoagulated blood and are spun in a centrifuge under standard conditions for a fixed period. The PCV is defined as the height of the column of packed red cells expressed as a fraction of the total height of the column of packed cells plus plasma. Automated blood counting machines calculate the PCV using red cell volume data and the red cell count.

The reference range is 0.40–0.51 for men and 0.36–0.48 for women.

Red cell count

The manual method for counting red cells involves diluting blood 1:200 in a solution containing formaldehyde and trisodium citrate (formol citrate) and filling a Neubauer, or similar type of counting chamber, with the diluted blood. The chamber is placed on the stage of a microscope and at least 500 RBCs are counted visually. RBCs determined from a total count of 500 cells are relatively imprecise; the precision of the count may be increased by counting larger number of cells.

Modern electronic blood-cell counters are capable of determining RBCs precisely and rapidly by counting large number of cells in a highly diluted sample of blood.

Estimation of red cell indices

The MCV, MCH and MCHC may be calculated from the Hb, PCV and RBC, determined by manual methods according to the following equations:

$$MCV\ (fL) = \frac{PCV\ (expressed\ as\ a\ fraction)}{RBC\ (L^{-1})} \times 10^{15}$$

$$MCH\ (pg) = \frac{Hb\ (g/dL)}{RBC\ (L^{-1})} \times 10^{13}$$

$$MCHC\ (g/dL) = \frac{Hb\ (g/dL)}{PCV\ (expressed\ as\ a\ fraction)}$$

Since RBCs obtained by manual methods are imprecise, both the MCV and MCH determined in this way are also unreliable; the only index that can be calculated reliably is the MCHC.

Electronic cell counters vary in their method of estimating the RBC and red cell size (i.e. MCV). The Coulter counters estimate these parameters on the basis of a change in electrical impedance when individual cells pass through a narrow orifice, the extent of the change being proportional to size. Other counters (e.g. Technicon) estimate the red cell count and MCV on the basis of the scattering of a focused beam of light when an individual cell passes through it. Thus, electronic cell counters in current use obtain a value for MCV by measurement rather than by calculation. All of them determine the PCV from the cell volume data and the RBC. The MCH and MCHC are calculated using the previous equations.

Electronic counters have to be standardized either with blood samples in which the various haematological parameters have been determined using reference methods, or with calibrants provided by the manufacturers. Although such counters have greatly improved the precision of all measurements (i.e. have considerably increased reproducibility), the accuracy of the MCV and MCHC determined by some such instruments (i.e. the relation between the observed result and the true value) is poor, particularly in the case of abnormal red cells.

Reference ranges in adults are given below as are common conditions in which abnormal values may be found.

Mean cell volume

The reference range is 82–99 fL (femtolitres). Values below this range are found in iron deficiency, thalassaemia syndromes and, sometimes, in the anaemia of chronic disorders. Values above the reference range are found in chronic alcoholism, vitamin B_{12} deficiency and folate deficiency.

Mean cell haemoglobin

The reference range is 27–33 pg (picograms). Values below this range are found in iron deficiency, thalassaemia syndromes and in some cases of anaemia in chronic diseases.

Mean cell haemoglobin concentration

The reference range is 32–36 g/dL. Its main use is in the diagnosis of iron deficiency. A low MCHC is a sensitive indicator of iron deficiency only when it is calculated using a PCV determined by the haematocrit method, or when it is obtained from a Technicon H1 series automated cell counter. It is not a sensitive indicator of iron deficiency when obtained from a Coulter counter since under these circumstances MCHC values only fall consistently below normal when the Hb is below 7 g/dL.

In apparently normal children between the ages of about 6 months and 15 years, the average values for the MCV and MCH are lower than in adults. At one time this was thought to be entirely due to a high prevalence of iron deficiency in children, but it is now clear that children with adequate iron stores have microcytic red cells and a low MCH (by adult standards) as an intrinsic feature of erythropoiesis in childhood. In children aged 1–8 years, the reference ranges for the MCV and MCH are, respectively, 70–88 fL and 24–30 pg. There is a gradual rise in the indices from the time of their lowest values at about 6 months of age; adult values are reached shortly after puberty.

White cell count

The manual method for determining the concentration of white cells in blood involves making a suitable dilution of whole blood, filling a counting chamber with the diluted blood and counting the white cells visually using a microscope. The diluting fluid contains acetic acid, which lyses the red cells, and a dye, such as gentian violet, to stain the white cells. This method has been superseded by electronic counting methods that are more precise, more accurate and much quicker. In these methods, the white cells are counted, after lysing the red cells, using the same principles as for red cell counting (i.e. by measurement of electrical impedance or light scattering).

Platelet count

Several manual methods are available. These involve making a suitable dilution of whole blood, filling a counting chamber and counting the unstained platelets using a phase-contrast microscope. A diluting fluid that has been found to work well is formaldehyde in sodium citrate (formol citrate). In one method, instead of diluting whole blood, platelet-rich plasma obtained by allowing the blood to settle at room temperature is diluted; this eliminates most of the red cells from the counting chamber. Electronic methods are now available that count platelets far more quickly and with far greater precision than the manual methods. The reference range for the platelet count is 160–450 × 10^9/L. Fully automated cell counters often count red cells and platelets in the same channel, distinguishing between them on the basis of size.

Reticulocyte count

Reticulocytes present in blood are red cells recently delivered from the marrow and contain remains of the RNA used in haemoglobin synthesis. The reticulocyte count is the best easily determined estimate that we have of the rate of production of viable red cells (p. 27). In the manual method for determining the reticulocyte count, the RNA is demonstrated by adding red cells to a solution of a dye such as brilliant cresyl blue, which precipitates the RNA as granules and filaments and also stains the precipitates. A film is then made on a slide and the proportion of reticulocytes to total red cells estimated by microscopy. When the rate of red cell production is normal, the count in adults is about 0.5–3.0%.

It is more useful to express the reticulocyte count as the absolute concentration per litre of blood than as a percentage since, when expressed as a percentage, the value is influenced by the red cell count (or Hb). For instance, a value of 6% with an Hb of 14 g/dL would correspond to the same absolute reticulocyte count as a value of 12% with an Hb of 7 g/dL. In normal adults, the absolute reticulocyte count determined by microscopy varies between 20 and 100 × 10^9/L.

Automated methods of reticulocyte counting are available in which the reticulocyte RNA is stained with a fluorescent dye such as acridine orange, thioflavin-T, thiazol orange or auramine O, and the reticulocytes are enumerated using fluorescence-activated flow cytometry. Automated methods are much more accurate and reproducible than the old manual method but the cells recognized by the two approaches are not identical.

Preparation and Romanowsky staining of blood or bone marrow smears

A small drop of blood or marrow aspirate is placed on the surface of a glass slide, near one end. Another slide (spreading slide) is placed in front of the drop at an angle of about 30° and is moved back slightly so that the drop spreads at the angle between the slides. The smear is then made by rapidly moving the spreading slide forward over the surface of the first slide. The smears are air dried and, except when required for certain cytochemical studies, fixed in methanol. The most commonly used stains for routine morphological studies include the May–Grünwald–Giemsa (MGG) stain, Wright's stain or Leishman's stain. These stains are collectively described as Romanowsky stains and contain eosin and methylene blue (plus derivatives of methylene blue such as various azure dyes).

Differential leucocyte count

In order to determine the relative proportion of neutrophil granulocytes, lymphocytes, etc. in the peripheral blood, their percentage distribution on a stained film is determined, assessing a minimum of 200 consecutive nucleated cells. The method is not very accurate as the distribution of various cell types on a film is not random: neutrophil granulocytes and monocytes predominate at the margins and tail of the film, and lymphocytes in the centre. Fortunately, when significant deviations from normality occur in patients they are greater than the error of the differential count.

From the total WBC and the differential leucocyte count, the concentration of various types of white cell per unit volume of blood (absolute counts) can be calculated. In adults, the upper limit of the reference range is usually taken to be 11 × 10^9/L of whole blood for the total white cell count, 7.5 × 10^9/L for neutrophil granulocytes and 3.5 × 10^9/L for lymphocytes.

A number of fully automated cell counters provide automated differential counts, using electrical impedance data or a combination of light scatter, cytochemical and other data to subclassify leucocytes.

Serum vitamin B$_{12}$ and red cell folate assays

In the past, serum vitamin B$_{12}$ and red cell folate levels were estimated microbiologically as the organisms *Lactobacillus leishmanii* and *Lactobacillus casei* require B$_{12}$ and folate, respectively, for growth and reproduction. The organism was incubated in the presence of serum or a haemolysate and the extent of growth estimated by the increase in turbidity, which is proportional to the amount of vitamin present. Microbiological assays are labour intensive and prone to periodic failure. Therefore, most laboratories now measure B$_{12}$ and folate levels using competitive protein-binding assays. These are based on the ability of ^{57}Co-labelled B$_{12}$ or ^{125}I-labelled pteroylglutamic acid (or these vitamins labelled with non-radioactive compounds) to compete with the corresponding vitamin in serum or a haemolysate, respectively, for combination with a specific vitamin-binding protein. Purified porcine intrinsic factor is used to bind B$_{12}$ and a bovine milk protein is used to bind folate. Several non-automated B_{12} and folate assay kits based on competitive protein binding are available. In addition there are some fully automated assays based on this principle and many laboratories in the UK use such a method. The reference ranges for the serum vitamin B_{12} and red cell folate levels are different for different assay methods.

Marrow aspiration and trephine biopsy of the marrow

A sample of marrow may be obtained for examination by aspiration from the iliac crest. After injecting a local anaesthetic into the skin and periosteum overlying the proposed site of aspiration, a special needle (with a stylet) is pushed through the bone into the marrow cavity. The stylet is then removed, a syringe fitted to the needle and the marrow aspirated. Drops of the aspirate are placed on glass slides and smeared. Some methanol-fixed smears are stained by a Romanowsky method and used to determine the cellularity of the marrow fragments (see Figs 3.2 and 14.1), the myeloid: erythroid ratio (p. 27) and the percentage distribution of the various cell types present. Others must always be stained for haemosiderin using Perls' acid ferrocyanide method (Prussian blue reaction), in order to assess: (i) iron stores within marrow fragments (i.e. the quantity of stainable iron present within macrophages; see Figs 4.5, 4.6 and 4.9); and (ii) the number, size and distribution of iron-containing granules within erythroblasts (see Fig. 4.7). Haemosiderin stains deep blue.

Another method of obtaining marrow for study is by trephine biopsy of the iliac crest, usually the posterior superior iliac spine. Here a special needle is used to obtain a core of bone and marrow. The specimen is fixed, decalcified and embedded in paraffin. Alternatively, the fixed core may be embedded in plastic without decalcification. Histological sections are prepared and stained with haematoxylin and eosin, Giemsa stain, Perls' acid ferrocyanide reaction for haemosiderin and, when appropriate, other stains. Some sections must always be stained by a silver impregnation method to study the distribution and quantity of reticulin fibres; this stain is important for the detection of myelofibrosis (see p. 131 and Fig. 12.7). Unlike marrow smears, histological sections allow the study of intercellular relationships and are therefore especially useful in detecting granulomas and focal accumulations of malignant cells.

Summary of reference ranges

The reference ranges (95% reference limits) for various haematological measurements in healthy adults are shown in Table 17.1.

Table 17.1 Reference ranges for Caucasian adults.

Haemoglobin	
Males	13.0–17.0 g/dL
Females (non-pregnant)	12.0–15.5 g/dL
Females (pregnant)	11.0–14.0 g/dL
Packed cell volume	
Males	0.40–0.51
Females	0.36–0.48
Red cell count	
Males	$4.4\text{–}5.8 \times 10^{12}/L$
Females	$4.1\text{–}5.2 \times 10^{12}/L$
Mean cell volume	82–99 fL
Mean cell haemoglobin	27–33 pg
Mean cell haemoglobin concentration	32–36 g/dL
White cell count	$4\text{–}11 \times 10^9/L$
Platelets	$160\text{–}450 \times 10^9/L$
Reticulocytes	$20\text{–}100 \times 10^9/L$
Serum iron	10–30 μmol/L
Serum transferrin	1.7–3.4 g/L
Serum ferritin	20–300 μg/L

Notes: dL — decilitre (100 mL); fL — femtolitre (1×10^{-15} L); pg — picogram (1×10^{-12} g); μ — micro (10^{-6}).

Chapter 18

Further Reading

General reference books

Greer J.P., Foerster J., Lukens J.N., Rodgers G.M., Paraskevas F., Glader B.E. (2003) *Wintrobe's Clinical Hematology*, 11th edn, Vols 1 and 2, Williams & Wilkins, Baltimore.

Hoffbrand A.V., Catovsky D., Tuddenham E.G.D. (eds) (2005) *Postgraduate Haematology*, 5th edn, Blackwell Publishing, Oxford.

Hoffman R., Benz E.J., Shattil S.J., Furie B., Cohen M.J., Silberstein L.E., McGlove P. (2005) *Hematology: Basic Principles and Practice*, 4th edn, Churchill Livingstone, Philadelphia.

Lichtman M.A., Beutler E., Kaushansky K., Kipps T.J., Seligsohn U., Prchal J. (2005) *William's Hematology*, 7th edn, McGraw-Hill, New York.

Nathan D.G., Orkin S.H., Ginsburg D., Look A.T. (2003) *Nathan and Oski's Hematology of Infancy and Childhood*, 6th edn, Elsevier Saunders, Philadelphia.

Wickramasinghe S.N., McCullough J. (eds) (2003) *Blood and Bone Marrow Pathology*, Elsevier Science Ltd., Edinburgh.

Chapter 1

Guo Y., Lubbert M., Engelhardt M. (2003) CD34-hematopoietic stem cells: current concepts and controversies. *Stem Cell.* **21**, 15–20.

Lecture Notes: Haematology, by NC Hughes-Jones, SN Wickramsinghe, CSR Hatton © 2008 Blackwell Publishing, ISBN: 9781405180504

Hermine O., Romeo P.-H. (2006) Regulation of erythropoiesis. In: C. Beaumont, P. Beris, Y. Beuzard, C. Brugnara (eds), *Disorders of Iron Homeostasis, Erythrocytes, Erythropoiesis*, European School of Haematology, pp. 39–70.

Higgs D.R., Weatherall D.J. (eds) (1993) The haemoglobinopathies. *Baillière's Clin. Haematol.* **6**(1), Baillière Tindall, London.

Hsia C.C.W. (1998) Respiratory function of hemoglobin. *N. Engl. J. Med.* **338**, 239–47.

Metcalf D. (2000) *Summon Up the Blood — in Dogged Pursuit of the Blood Cell Regulators*, Alpha Med Press, Dayton, OH.

Metcalf D., Nicola N.A. (1995) *The Haemopoietic Colony Stimulating Factors*, Cambridge University Press, Cambridge.

Verfaillie C. (2003) Regulation of hematopoiesis. In: S.N. Wickramasinghe, J. McCullough (eds), *Blood and Bone Marrow Pathology*, Elsevier Science Ltd., Edinburgh, pp. 71–85.

Whetton A.D. (ed.) (1997) Molecular haemopoiesis. *Baillière's Clin. Haematol.* **10**, 429–619.

Wickramasinghe S.N. (2007) Bone marrow. In: S.E. Mills (ed.), *Histology for Pathologists*, 3rd edn, Lippincott Williams & Wilkins, Philadelphia, pp. 799–836.

Chapter 2

McMullin M.F., Bareford D., Campbell P., Green A.R., Harrison C., Hunt B., Oscier D., Polkey M.I.,

Reilly J.T., Rosenthal E., Ryan K., Pearson T.C., Wilkins B.; General Haematology Task Force of the British Committee for Standards in Haematology (2005).Guidelines for the diagnosis, investigation and management of polycythaemia/erythrocytosis. *Br. J. Haematol.* **130**, 174–95.

Messinezy M., van der Walt J.D., Pearson T.C. (2003) Polycythemia (the erythrocytoses). In: S.N. Wickramasinghe, J. McCullough (eds), *Blood and Bone Marrow Pathology*, Elsevier Science Ltd., Edinburgh, pp. 283–95.

Pearson T.C. (1991) Apparent polycythaemia. *Blood Rev.* **5**, 205–13.

Souid A.K., Dubansky A.S., Richman P., Sadowitz P.D. (1993) Polycythemia: a review article and case report of erythrocytosis secondary to Wilm's tumor. *Pediatr. Hematol. Oncol.* **10**, 215–21.

Territo M.C., Rosove M.H. (1991) Cyanotic congenital heart disease: hematologic management. *J. Am. Coll. Cardiol.* **18**, 320–22.

Chapter 3

Beutler E. (1996) Glucose-6-phosphate-dehydrogenase population genetics and clinical manifestations. *Blood Rev.* **10**, 45–52.

Bolton-Maggs P.H., Stevens R.F., Dodd N.J., Lamont G., Tittensor P., King M.J.; General Haematology Task Force of the British Committee for Standards in Haematology (2004). Guidelines for the diagnosis and management of hereditary spherocytosis. *Br. J. Haematol.* **126**, 455–74.

Dacie J.V. (1985) *The Haemolytic Anaemias*, 3rd edn, Vol 1: *The Hereditary Haemolytic Anaemias*, Part 1. Churchill Livingstone, Edinburgh.

Dacie J.V. (1988) *The Haemolytic Anaemias*, 3rd edn, Vol 2: *The Hereditary Haemolytic Anaemias*, Part 2. Churchill Livingstone, Edinburgh.

Dacie J.V. (1992) *The Haemolytic Anaemias*, 3rd edn, Vol 3: *The Auto-Immune Haemolytic Anaemias*. Churchill Livingstone, Edinburgh.

Delaunay J. (2007) The molecular basis of hereditary red cell membrane disorders. *Blood Rev.* **21**, 1–20.

Delaunay J., Cartron J.-P. (2006) Disorders of the red cell membrane. In: C. Beaumont, P. Beris, Y. Beuzard, C. Brugnara (eds), *Disorders of Iron Homeostasis, Erythrocytes, Erythropoiesis*, European School of Haematology, pp. 364–90.

Engelfriet C.P., Overbeeke M.A., von dem Borne A.E. (1992) Autoimmune hemolytic anemia. *Semin. Hematol.* **29**, 3–12.

Galacteros F. (2006) Sickle cell disease: a short guide to management. In: C. Beaumont, P. Beris, Y. Beuzard, C. Brugnara (eds), *Disorders of Iron Homeostasis, Erythrocytes, Erythropoiesis*, European School of Haematology, pp. 276–309.

Mehta A., Mason P.J., Vulliamy T.J. (2000) Glucose 6-phospate dehydrogenase deficiency. *Baillière's Clin. Haematol.* **13**, 21–38.

Sergeant G.R. (1992) *Sickle Cell Anaemia*, 2nd edn, Oxford University Press, Oxford.

Steinberg M.H., Forget B.G., Higgs D.R., Nagel R.L. (eds) (2001) *Disorders of Hemoglobin*, Cambridge University Press, Cambridge.

Steinberg M.H., Barton F., Castro O. *et al.* (2003) Effect of hydroxyurea on mortality and morbidity in adult sickle cell anemia: risks and benefits up to 9 years of treatment. *JAMA* **289**, 1645–51.

Tanner M.J.A., Anstee D.J. (eds) (1999) Red cell membrane disorders. *Baillière's Clin. Haematol.* **12**, 605–770.

Weatherall D. (2005) Beginnings: the molecular pathology of hemoglobin. In: D. Provan, J. Gribben (eds), *Molecular Hematology*, Blackwell Publishing, Oxford, pp. 1–17.

Weatherall D.J., Clegg J.B. (2001) *The Thalassaemia Syndromes*, 4th edn, Blackwell Science, Oxford.

Zanella A. (ed.) (2000) Inherited disorders of red cell metabolism. *Clin. Haematol.* **13**, 1–150.

Chapter 4

Andrews N.C. (1999) Disorders of iron metabolism. *N. Engl. J. Med.* **341**, 1986–95.

Andrews N.C. (2000) Iron metabolism and absorption. *Rev. Clin. Exp. Hematol.* **4**, 283–301.

Barton J.C., Edwards C.Q. (2000) *Hemochromatosis*, Cambridge University Press, Cambridge.

Beard J. (2003) Iron deficiency alters brain development and functioning. *J. Nutr.* **133**(5 Suppl 1), 1468S–72S.

Beaumont C., Vaulont S. (2006) Iron homeostasis. In: C. Beaumont, P. Beris, Y.Beuzard, C. Brugnara (eds),

Disorders of Iron Homeostasis, Erythrocytes, Erythropoiesis, European School of Haematology, pp. 392–406.

Feder J.N., Gnirke A., Thomas W. *et al.* (1996) A novel MHC class I-like gene is mutated in patients with hereditary haemochromatosis. *Nat. Genet.* **13**, 399–408.

Griffiths W.J. (2007) Review article: the genetic basis of haemochromatosis. *Aliment. Pharmacol. Ther.* **26**, 331–42.

Hallberg L., Bengtsson C., Lapidus L., Lindstedt G., Lundberg P.A., Hulten L. (1993) Screening for iron deficiency: an analysis based on bone-marrow examinations and serum ferritin determinations in a population sample of women. *Br. J. Haematol.* **85**, 787–98.

Hershko C. (ed.) (1994) Clinical disorders of iron metabolism. *Baillières Clin. Haematol.* **7**(4), Baillière Tindall, London.

Hershko C. (2006) Prevalence and causes of iron deficiency anaemia. In: C. Beaumont, P. Beris, Y. Beuzard, C. Brugnara (eds), *Disorders of Iron Homeostasis, Erythrocytes, Erythropoiesis*, European School of Haematology, pp. 408–19.

Krantz S.B. (1994) Pathogenesis and treatment of the anemia of chronic disease. *Am. J. Med. Sci.* **307**, 353–9.

Lansdown R., Wharton B.A. (1995) Iron and mental and motor behaviour in children. In: *Iron. Nutritional and Physiological Significance. Report of a British Nutrition Foundation Task Force*, Chapman and Hall, London, pp. 65–78.

May A., Bishop D.F. (1998) The molecular biology and pyridoxine responsiveness of X-linked sideroblastic anaemia. *Haematologica* **83**, 56–70.

Mills A.F. (1990) Surveillance for anaemia: risk factors in patterns of milk intake. *Arch. Dis. Child.* **65**, 428–31.

Pippard M.J. (2003) Iron-deficiency anemia, anemia of chronic disorders, and iron overload. In: S.N. Wickramasinghe, J. McCullough (eds), *Blood and Bone Marrow Pathology*, Elsevier Science Ltd., Edinburgh, pp. 203–28.

Sears D.A. (1992) Anemia of chronic disease. *Med. Clin. North. Am.* **76**, 567–79.

Sheard N.F. (1994) Iron deficiency and infant development. *Nutr. Rev.* **52**, 137–40.

Chapter 5

Carmel R. (1995) Malabsorption of food cobalamin. *Baillière's Clin. Hematol.* **8**, 639–55.

Carmel R. (ed.) (1999) Beyond megaloblastic anemia: new paradigms of cobalamin and folate deficiency. *Semin. Hematol.* **36**(1), 1–100.

Chanarin I. (1990) *The Megaloblastic Anaemias*, 3rd edn, Blackwell Scientific Publications, Oxford.

Glesson P.A., Toh B.H. (1991) Molecular targets in pernicious anaemia. *Immunol. Today* **12**, 233–8.

Healton E.H., Savage D.G., Brust J.C.M., Garrett T.J., Lindenbaum J. (1991) Neurologic aspects of cobalamin deficiency. *Medicine* **70**, 229–45.

Horton L., Coburn R.J., England J.M., Himsworth R.L. (1976) The haematology of hypothyroidism. *Q. J. Med.* **45**, 101–23.

Wickramasinghe S.N. (ed.) (1995) Megaloblastic anaemia. *Baillière's Clin. Haematol.* **8**(3), Baillière Tindall, London.

Wickramasinghe S.N. (1999) The wide spectrum and unresolved issues of megaloblastic anemia. *Semin. Hematol.* **36**, 3–18.

Wickramasinghe S.N. (2006) Diagnosis of megaloblastic anaemias. *Blood Rev.* **20**, 299–318.

Wickramasinghe S.N., Corridan B., Hasan R., Marjot D.H. (1994) Correlations between acetaldehyde-modified haemoglobin, carbohydrate-deficient transferrin (CDT) and haematological abnormalities in chronic alcoholism. *Alcohol Alcohol.* **29**, 415–23.

Chapter 6

Bain B.J. (2000) Hypereosinophilia. *Curr. Opin. Hematol.* **7**, 21–5.

Beeson P.B., Bass D.A. (1977) *The Eosinophil*, W.B. Saunders, Philadelphia.

Callan M.F. (2003) The evolution of antigen-specific CD8 T cell responses after natural primary infection of humans with Epstein–Barr virus. *Viral Immunol.* **16**, 3–16.

Chetham M.M., Roberts K.B. (1991) Infectious mononucleosis in adolescents. *Pediatr. Ann.* **20**, 206–13.

Connelly K.P., DeWitt L.D. (1994) Neurologic complications of infectious mononucleosis. *Pediatr. Neurol.* **10**, 181–4.

Liesveld J.L., Abboud C.N. (1992) Hypereosinophilic syndromes: an update. *Int. J. Clin. Lab. Res.* **22**, 5–10.

Mahmoud A.A.F., Austen K.F., Simon A.S. (1980) *The Eosinophil in Health and Disease*, Grune & Stratton, New York.

Okano M. (2000) Haematological associations of Epstein–Barr virus infection. *Bailliere's Clin. Haematol.* **13**, 199–214.

Peterson L., Hrisinko M.A. (1993) Benign lymphocytosis and reactive neutrophilia. Laboratory features provide diagnostic clues. *Clin. Lab. Med.* **13**, 863–77.

Chapters 7–13

References are provided to papers on microarray gene expression profiling and imatinib as these are two of the most significant advances in the field of hematological malignancies in recent years. The WHO classification reference book[*] Jaffe E.S. *et al.* provides a very clear concise reference for all the hematological malignancies and related disorders, and is highly recommended to those students of hematology who require greater detail particularly with regard to the pathology and genetics of the disorders.

Attal M., Harousseau J.L., Stoppa A.M. *et al.* (1996) A prospective, randomized trial of autologous bone marrow transplantation and chemotherapy in multiple myeloma. Intergroupe Francais du Myelome. *N. Engl. J. Med.* **335**(2), 91–7.

Cavenagh J.D., Oakervee H., UK Myeloma Forum and the BCSH Haematology/Oncology Task Forces (2003). Thalidomide in multiple myeloma: current status and future prospects. *Br. J. Haematol.* **120**(1), 18–26.

Grimwade D., Walker H., Oliver F. *et al.* (1998) The importance of diagnostic cytogenetics on outcome in AML: analysis of 1,612 patients entered into the MRC AML 10 trial. The Medical Research Council Adult and Children's Leukaemia Working Parties. *Blood* **92**(7), 2322–33. [Comment: *Blood* (2000) **96**(5), p. 2002.]

Hancock B.W., Selby P., MacLennan K.A., Armitage, J.O. (2000) The origin of B-cell lymphomas in relation to the structure and function of lymphoid tissue. In: *Malignant Lymphoma*, Arnold, London.

[*]Jaffe E.S., Harris N.L.,Vardiman J.W. (2001) Pathology and genetics of tumours of the haemopoietic system and tissues. *WHO Classification of Tumours*, Vol. 3. World Health Organization.

Kuppers R., Klein U., Hansmann M.L., Rajewsky K. (1999) Cellular origin of human B-cell lymphomas. *N. Engl. J. Med.* **341**(20), 1520–9.

Mauch P.M., Armitage J.O., Diehl V., Hoppe R.T., Weiss L.M. (eds) (1999) *Hodgkin's Disease*, Lippincott Williams and Wilkins, Philadelphia.

Rosenwald A., Wright G., Chan W.C. *et al.* (2002) The use of molecular profiling to predict survival after chemotherapy for diffuse large-B-cell lymphoma. *N. Engl. J. Med.* **346**(25), 1937–47.

Savage D.G., Antman K.H. (2002) Imatinib mesylate — a new oral targeted therapy. *N. Engl. J. Med.* **346**, 683–93.

Schwartz R.S. (2003) Shattuck lecture: diversity of the immune repertoire and immunoregulation. *N. Engl. J. Med.* **348**, 1017–26.

Slavin S., Nagler A., Naparstek E. *et al.* (1998) Nonmyeloablative stem cell transplantation and cell therapy as an alternative to conventional bone marrow transplantation with lethal cytoreduction for the treatment of malignant and nonmalignant hematologic diseases. *Blood* **91**(3), 756–63.

Tefferi A. (2000) Myelofibrosis with myeloid metaplasia. *N. Engl. J. Med.* **342**, 1255–65.

Chapter 14

Alter B.P. (1993) Fanconi's anaemia and its variability. *Br. J. Haematol.* **85**, 9–14.

Bacigalupo A. (2007) Aplastic anemia: pathogenesis and treatment. *Hematology — Am. Soc. Hematol. Educ. Program.*, 23–8.

Brown K.E. (2000) Haematological consequences of parvovirus B19 infection. *Baillière's Clin. Haematol.* **13**, 245–59.

Dessypris E.N. (1991) The biology of pure red cell aplasia. *Semin. Hematol.* **28**, 275–84.

Dianzani I., Garelli E., Ramenghi U. (1996) Diamond-Blackfan anemia: a congenital defect in erythropoiesis. *Haematologica* **81**, 560–72.

Dokal I. (2006) Fanconi's anaemia and related bone marrow failure syndromes. *Br. Med. Bull.* **77–78**, 37–53.

Fisch P., Handgretinger R., Schaefer H.E. (2000) Pure red cell aplasia. *Br. J. Haematol.* **111**, 1010–22.

Gazda H.T., Sieff C.A. (2006) Recent insights into the pathogenesis of Diamond-Blackfan anaemia. *Br. J. Haematol.* **135**, 149–57.

Gordon-Smith E.C. (2003) Aplastic anemia: acquired and inherited. In: S.N. Wickramasinghe, J. McCullough (eds), *Blood and Bone Marrow Pathology*, Elsevier Science Ltd., Edinburgh, pp. 249–63.

Gordon-Smith E.C., Issaragrisil S. (1992) Epidemiology of aplastic anaemia. *Baillière's Clin. Haematol.* **5**(2), 475–91.

Willig T.-N., Draptchinskaia N., Dianzani I. *et al.* (1999) Mutations in ribosomal protein S19 gene and Diamond Blackfan anemia: wide variations in phenotypic expression. *Blood* **94**, 4294–306.

Young N.S., Abkowitz J.L., Luzzatto L. (2000) New insights into the pathophysiology of acquired cytopenias. *Hematology — Am. Soc. Hematol. Educ. Program.*, 18–38.

Young N.S., Calado R.T., Scheinberg P. (2006) Current concepts in the pathophysiology and treatment of aplastic anemia. *Blood* **108**, 2509–19.

Chapter 15

Astermark J., Donfield S.M., DiMichele D.M., Gringeri A., Gilbert S.A., Waters J., Berntorp E., for the FENOC Study Group (2007). A randomized comparison of bypassing agents in hemophilia complicated by an inhibitor: the FEIBA NovoSeven Comparative (FENOC) Study. *Blood* **109**, 546–51.

Bowden D.J. (2002) Haemophilia A and haemophilia B: molecular insights. *Mol. Pathol.* **55**, 1–18.

Cines D.B., Bussel J.B. (2005) How I treat idiopathic thrombocytopenic purpura (ITP). *Blood* **106**, 2244–51.

Colman R.W., Marder V.J., Clowes A.W., George J.N., Goldhaber S.Z. (2005) *Hemostasis and Thrombosis: Basic Principles and Clinical Practice*, 5th edn, Lipincott Williams & Wilkins, Hagerstown.

Crowther M.A., Kelton J.G. (2003) Congenital thrombophilic states associated with venous thrombosis: a qualitative overview and proposed classification system. *Ann. Intern. Med.* **138**, 128–34.

Dahlbäck B. (2005) Blood coagulation and its regulation by anticoagulant pathways: genetic pathogenesis of bleeding and thrombotic diseases. *J. Intern. Med.* **257**, 209–23.

George J.N. (2000) Platelets. *Lancet* **355**, 1531–9.

George J.N. (2006a) Management of patients with refractory immune thrombocytopenic purpura. *J. Thromb. Haemost.* **4**, 1664–72.

George J.N. (2006b) Clinical practice. Thrombotic thrombocytopenic purpura. *N. Engl. J. Med.* **354**, 1927–35.

Guidelines on oral anticoagulation (warfarin), 3rd edition — 2005 update: Baglin T.P., Keeling D.M., Watson H.G. (2006) *Br. J. Haematol.* **132**, 277–85.

Guidelines on the investigation and management of the antiphospholipid syndrome (2000) *Br. J. Haematol.* **109**, 704–15.

Hirsh J., O'Donnell M., Eikelboom J.W. (2007) Beyond unfractionated heparin and warfarin: current and future advances. *Circulation* **116**, 552–60.

Kelton J.G., Bussel J.B. (2000) Idiopathic thrombocytopenic purpura. *Semin. Hematol.* **37**, 219–314.

Lane D.A., Grant P.J. (2000) Role of hemostatic gene polymorphisms in venous and arterial thrombotic disease. *Blood* **95**, 1517–32.

Lee C.A. (2003) Inherited disorders of coagulation. In: S.N. Wickramasinghe, J. McCullough (eds), *Blood and Bone Marrow Pathology*, Elsevier Science Ltd., Edinburgh, pp. 557–75.

Li X., Swisher K.K., Vesely S.K., George J.N. (2007) Drug-induced thrombocytopenia: an updated systematic review, 2006. *Drug Saf.* **30**, 185–6.

Lilleyman J. (2000) Chronic childhood idiopathic thrombocytopenic purpura. *Baillière's Clin. Haematol.* **13**, 469–83.

MacCallum P.K., Meade T.W. (eds) (1999) Thrombophilia. *Baillière's Clin. Haematol.* **12**, 329–603.

Mannucci P.M. (2001) How I treat patients with von Willebrand disease. *Blood* **97**, 1915–19.

Mannucci P.M., Peyvandi F. (2007) TTP and ADAMTS13: When is testing appropriate? *Am. Soc. Hematol. Educ. Program.* 121–6.

Moake J.L. (2002) Thrombotic thrombocytopenic purpura and the hemolytic uremic syndrome. *Arch. Pathol. Lab. Med.* **126**, 1430–3.

Watts R.G. (2004) Idiopathic thrombocytopenic purpura: a 10-year natural history study at the children's hospital of Alabama. *Clin. pediatr.* **43**, 691–702.

Chapter 16

Barbara J.A.J., Regan F.A.M., Contreras M.C. (2008) *Transfusion Microbiology*. Cambridge University Press, Cambridge.

Brennan M.T., Barbara J.A.J. (1993) Transfusion-transmitted disease. *Curr. Opin. Hematol.* **1A**, 320–9.

Contreras M. (ed.) (1998) *ABC of Transfusion*, 3rd edn, BMJ Publications Group, London.

Dodd R.Y. (2007) Current risk for transfusion transmitted infections. *Curr. Opin. Hematol.* **14**, 671–6.

Klein H.G., Anstee D.J. (2005) Mollison's *Blood Transfusion in Clinical Medicine*, 11th edn, Blackwell Publishing, Oxford.

Leikola J. (1993) Viral risks of blood transfusion. *Rev. Med. Microbiol.* **4**, 32–9.

McCullough J. (2004) *Transfusion Medicine*, 2nd edn, Churchill Livingstone, New York.

Murphy M.F., Pamphilon D.H. (eds) (2005) *Practical Transfusion Medicine*, 2nd edn, Blackwell Publishing, Oxford.

Regan F., Taylor C. (2002) Recent developments. Blood transfusion medicine. *Br. Med. J.* **325**, 143–7.

Chapter 17

Lewis S.M., Bain B.J., Bates I. (2006) *Dacie & Lewis Practical Haematology*, 10th edn, Elsevier, Philadelphia.

Index

Page numbers in *italics* refer to figures and those in **bold** to tables, but note that figures and tables are only indicated when they are separated from their text references. Index entries are filed in letter-by-letter alphabetical order.